PASTORAL CARE TO THE CANCER PATIENT

PASTORAL CARE TO THE CANCER PATIENT

By

THE REVEREND NANCY VAN DYKE PLATT

Chaplain and Oncology Resident
Rush-Presbyterian-St. Luke's Hospital
Chicago, Illinois
Priest Assistant
Bishop Anderson House
Chicago, Illinois

Foreword by

The Rev. Christian A. Hovde

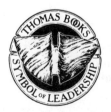

CHARLES C THOMAS • PUBLISHER
Springfield • Illinois • U.S.A.

Published and Distributed Throughout the World by

CHARLES C THOMAS ● PUBLISHER

Bannerstone House

301-327 East Lawrence Avenue, Springfield, Illinois, U.S.A.

© *1980, by* CHARLES C THOMAS ● PUBLISHER

ISBN 0-398-04051-6

Library of Congress Catalog Card Number: 80-15813

With THOMAS BOOKS *careful attention is given to all details of
manufacturing and design. It is the Publisher's desire to present books that
are satisfactory as to their physical qualities and artistic possibilities and
appropriate for their particular use.* THOMAS BOOKS *will be true to those
laws of quality that assure a good name and good will.*

Printed in the United States of America
V-R-1

Library of Congress Cataloging in Publication Data

Platt, Nancy Van Dyke.
   Pastoral care to the cancer patient.

   Bibliography: p.
   1. Pastoral medicine. 2. Cancer patients.
I. Title.
BV4335.P567   253   80-15813
ISBN 0-398-04051-6

To the strangers who became friends
as they shared their lives and deaths with me.

FOREWORD

PROFESSIONAL literature almost always contains ideas couched in technical language and used within the science as the basis either of teaching or of study that are never translated into the popular genre. Only occasionally do some of these ideas or techniques find their way out of the technical jungle and are found to be useful and illuminating in a larger or more popular sense by persons not intimately concerned with the sciences in which they originated. One of these is the "verbatim report" and the analysis of the data contained within it.

The verbatim report is the recording on paper, to the best of the reporter's ability to remember the entire event, of the total conversation between two people. It usually is centered around a specific event in a long series of such conversations and connected with very stressful or anxiety producing circumstances such as the death of a loved one, or even one's own impending demise; the threat of physical damage implicit in radical surgery or the implications of increasing dependency or isolation resulting from relentless disability or old age.

The reporter's ability to remember the event, and the analysis of the data contained in the report, form the basis for an understanding of the fears, coping mechanisms, strengths, and unrecognized blind spots in both the reporter and the person with whom he or she is talking. The technique is used extensively in the process of clinical pastoral education as a way of showing students what they are or not accomplishing in the attempt to aid someone in trouble or distress. Often the student finds that because of his own blind spots he has not recognized a cry for help or a clue to the actual point of distress in the patient. People in trouble often cannot articulate exactly where it hurts or why the hurt is so strongly felt when the injury appears slight or should be seen as normal occurrence. When the student harbors fears of his own related to the same type of injury or does not understand that he has those fears, he fails to recognize or rejects the same feelings in others and is therefore of no help to them.

Persons reveal more of their inner feelings and fears by their indirect responses in conversation than by their direct statements. Analysis of the entire conversation provides a way of seeing the pattern of the response rather than the words of the responses. The pattern is often more revealing than the exact words used. Indirection and talking around the point rather than to the point are ways of avoiding the pain of exposure and at the same time provide a way of allowing an acute observer to see what the trouble may be.

In the material that follows, the author has attempted to show this process both as illustration of the process itself and as concrete examples of specific problems faced by human beings in trouble. In part, these examples are both process and analysis, since they obviously do not include the entire conversation in any one example. Some judgement upon the worth of any set of statements in any example had to be made, and the text that accompanies the sample conversations reveals both the biases of the author and the ability of the author to correctly assess the core of the problem.

It should be pointed out that the process is one that requires some degree of skill derived from repeated attempts to record and then to analyze the record and depends a great deal on a third party who aids by dispassionately looking at both sides of the conversation at the same time and pointing out the missed cues or evasions, tying them to the larger issues of the circumstances in which the event took place.

Careful examination of the materials that follow will reveal a good deal about the process. One can, and probably should, quarrel with some of the conclusions drawn in specific examples, but the fact that use is made of this process in attempting to describe in a coherent manner a host of related problems is an important contribution to an understanding of the peculiar issues related to cancer and its consequences in the entire living situation for both patient and family.

One of the things now recognized in the field of counseling

is the importance of the maintenance of a feeling of control of his or her circumstances by the patient. All of us find it more simple or easy to prescribe a course of action or understanding for someone else than to provide an atmosphere or environment in which that person can see and claim alternatives acceptable to himself. We have difficulty with the time, patience, and energy expenditure necessary to facilitate the other person's decision making. We like to make the decisions ourselves and expect others to accept them as their own. Unfortunately, human behavior rarely works this way, and the patient who apparently adopts our decisions may actually be thereby unable to use his own resources to heal himself or to carve out a new way of existing acceptable to himself. Without such personal work, successfully completed to some degree, no one survives catastrophe for long. The support given by other people should never be of such nature as to remove the personal feeling of independence and responsibility of the patient.

The final section of the material advances the thesis that a constructive attitude about one's own integrity and worth rather than a destructively critical attitude may have a direct biological effect on the ability of any person to mobilize his own resources to fight a disease or its consequences. This is not a new idea; it has been voiced before as the "will to live," the need to survive, and the ability to overcome apparently insuperable obstacles. It has been only in recent years, however, that this idea has been supported by research and documentation of both the theological and biological sciences. The data are admittedly weak at the moment, but there is promise that a direct relationship may be found linking the ability to think well of one's self with the ability of one's body to call up the defenses needed for survival of any kind. The idea bears close attention and a great deal of further work.

Finally, the issues raised herein are the common yet critical ones in all human existence under difficult circumstances. The contribution made to the understanding of the issues is one of continuity, understanding of the basic needs for control and responsibility even in diminished physical strength, and the creation of the environment in which anyone can afford to live while undergoing acute physical distress or even death. If we counselors can afford to counsel rather than direct, our patients will be able to find within themselves the resources to do their own work and do it well. It is a truism that no one can do that work for them.

The Rev. Christian A. Hovde

ACKNOWLEDGMENTS

MINISTRY to cancer patients and their families is a shared ministry. I owe many thanks to those people who supported me ánd grieved with me during the years that I collected material for this book.

First of all my family, David, Jon, Elizabeth, and Tom, who listened to me grieve for people they met only through my eyes, and kept the household going when I stayed with other families. My supervisors, Rev. Bernard Pennington and Dr. Larry Ulrich, and my CPE peers shared my questions and problems with me and to them my gratitude.

Assistance in writing and preparation of this book were given me by David Moss, Howard Clinebell, and Christian Hovde. The Rev. Edward M. Copland assisted me with the parochial aspects of ministry to cancer patients and their families.

Thanks also goes to Mrs. Sharon Steffen who patiently typed and retyped and to Mr. Sherwood K. Platt who provided me with a retreat for several summers in which I wrote this book.

My appreciation to Amelia Barbus and Carl and Stephanie Simonton for allowing me to use their material in this book.

CONTENTS

The Dying Person's Bill of Rights*

I have the right to be treated as a living human being until I die.

I have the right to maintain a sense of hopefulness however changing its focus may be.

I have the right to be cared for by those who can maintain a sense of hopefulness, however changing this might be.

I have the right to express my feelings and emotions about my approaching death in my own way.

I have the right to participate in decisions concerning my care.

I have the right to expect continuing medical and nursing attention even though cure goals must be changed to comfort goals.

I have the right not to die alone.

I have the right to have my questions answered honestly.

I have the right not to be deceived.

I have the right to have help from and for my family in accepting my death.

I have the right to die in peace and dignity.

I have the right to retain my individuality and not be judged for my decisions, which may be contrary to the beliefs of others.

I have the right to discuss and enlarge my religious and/or spiritual experiences, whatever these mean to others.

I have the right to expect that the sanctity of the human body will be respected after death.

I have the right to be cared for by sensitive, caring knowledgeable people who will attempt to understand my needs and will be able to gain some satisfaction in helping me face my death.

---

*Reprinted by permission of Amelia J. Barbus, who conducted the workshop at which this Bill of Rights was created. The workshop discussed "The Terminally Ill Patient and the Helping Person."

PASTORAL CARE TO
THE CANCER PATIENT

CHAPTER 1

THE CANCER PATIENT IN THE PARISH

CANCER creates a crisis of major proportions that wrecks financial, emotional, physical, and spiritual resources in a family or member of a parish. Depleted parishioners often need large amounts of support and care to function during their lengthy involvement with the vagaries of the disease. Whether cancer is cured or whether it kills, this time is experienced by all with feelings of helplessness and hopelessness.

The pastor who ministers to those parishioners who are involved in the crisis of cancer will have his own needs for support and the conservation of his energy as well. He is often looked to as the one "who understands what is going on," or who can talk to the doctor on a peer level. Yet in a lifetime, the pastor may deal with five to ten cancer patients and their families who have different diseases and varying degrees of success in treatment.

This manual on pastoral care to the cancer patient presents typical cases and problems encountered in the course of working with cancer patients. Moreover, whatever the words the pastor hears, the underlying concern has one of several basic foci and feelings of which he needs to be aware.

The following case study — the death of a young man from the viewpoint of his pastor who "entered in the middle," — presents an array of typical problems that most pastors would meet, but might deal with differently depending on their parishioner's circumstances. The pastor's reflections follow — his efforts both to learn from and detach from his involvement with the patient.

Case Study

P. J. was a forty-two-year-old, white, married male with a wife and one son. He worked for an advertising firm. He had

3

had cancer for three years, and there were several kinds of cancer. He had two surgical procedures, one of which left him almost blind, and several chemotherapy regimens, but there was little evidence of remission. He and more especially his wife and son had been members of the parish for several years before the parish pastor arrived; the patient lived a year and three to four months afterwards.

The pastor's first meeting with the patient was at a parish function when the patient, who used a long cane, was being helped into the room. Later, another parishioner, a friend of the patient, gave the pastor a brief history of the patient and his illness. He described the cohesion around the family during each crisis, and the prayer that accompanied the parish concern. The parishioner was amazed that the patient was alive.

The wife initiated the first contact with the pastor shortly thereafter. She felt that she was having trouble with her son because "he is not getting male attention"; she also stated that she needed counseling. She was referred to a family counselor who focused with her and her son upon the role shift that was taking place in the family. The wife would soon be the principal parent. Subsequently, other male parish members helped her with this role. As the patient became less mobile, they included his son in their own outside activities.

The wife initiated the second contact after the death of her father, which took place shortly after the first contact. "Why do these things have to happen?" she wondered. She was faced with the loss of two significant male support figures in her life. She saw the pastor on a regular basis after that, and the family began including the pastor and his family in their social activities.

The family interaction was somewhat strained. The wife felt that the patient was "giving in to pain and his own feelings." She tended to deny his blindness, "P. J.'s problem," and discomfort. The patient felt that his wife was "not a nurturing person, but very demanding," yet he had difficulty accepting help when he was walking. The couple together had a view of themselves as "winners." They tended to look at success in terms of a large home, more than they could presently afford. The patient bought diamond earrings for his wife, which he would pay for with future earnings. He saw himself as being president of his company one day. The son sporadically had problems in school.

Shortly after his birthday, the patient was hospitalized. His behavior during this hospitalization is the prototype of his efforts to control his illness and his situation. He was never subservient in the hospital and never entrusted his medical care to others. He kept a journal of intricate records of his treatments, his medications, and calls to the doctor, although his limited vision made this difficult. He was aware of all of his treatment, although his wife may not have been. He also asked only for what he absolutely needed and could not get for himself. He initiated occasional conversations about his own death and seemed to anticipate it on one level. He wished to die in control of his faculties, not in pain or overmedicated like a vegetable. His conversation would then shift to the future and his anxiety over leaving his son without male identifications. His son was brought by the pastor for visits in a private lounge area of the hospital as the patient wished.

While the pastor related to the rest of the family as a counselor, he became a friend to the patient. Discussion centered around anything but his disease. At times, however, the patient would initiate brief discussions about his own death. The pastor and his family were included in a holiday dinner. Although the patient was in pain, he contributed what he could to the gathering. The following holiday (Christmas) the pastor had a call from the wife. She initiated a visit to the patient's sister in the South "where it was warm," because she "needed to get out more." The sister was described by the patient as a "nurturing person." Upon their return, the patient became less mobile due to the weather and a medication change; he stayed home and did not go to work. His wife became increasingly angry because she felt he was "giving up."

In his last long hospitalization, the patient's requests for visits became almost daily. His wife spent short periods of time visiting and then went on expensive shopping sprees — an act of denial and a search for normalcy and relief. The son spent more and more time with friends and with his mother. School authorities were told of the situation and members of the parish helped foster the son's needs. His father talked to him on the phone, but did not "want him to see me in pain." The patient often asked the pastor to "come now" and the pastor played an active part in some nursing care, feeding the patient and "doing better than those at the hospital." Much of the time was spent in silence as the patient dozed or listened to music. Because the patient may not have been Episcopalian, there was no Communion. The patient requested only that "you pray for me at [a specific time, e.g. morning prayer]." The patient's wife came to Mass regularly. She initiated a discussion of the funeral plans, but the pastor asked her to wait to discuss them.

After a second surgical procedure to relieve the pain, the pastor and the patient's wife began keeping his journal for him. Other visitors were asked to come later if the pastor was visiting. There were no more conversations about life and death or the future. The patient would ask, "when are you coming tomorrow?" His life became a struggle against pain and "they," the hospital staff. The latter supported him in his rebellion and efforts to maintain his identity, yet there were times when they had to be firm with him. His wife begain to receive more of her medical information from the staff.

The patient "fired" his doctors and retained new ones who would try one more oncology "trick." Everyone hoped it would succeed, but success had come to be measured in terms of the future as "how can I manage the pain and the time left?"

After surgery, the patient was totally bedridden, although there was some reduction in pain. He told his wife to "make sure everyone has a good time" at his funeral, and his wife began to make concrete plans. He also wanted his wife to sit with him and hold his hand as he slipped in and out of a comatose state. She said in his hearing that she wished "he would die, that he didn't have to suffer so much," giving him "permission to die." She seemed to have accepted his death before he did, yet she roused him after he sank into deeper sleep.

Shortly before the patient died, the wife asked the priest to plan the music for the services, but the priest put this off. The hospital staff called the wife and the priest after the patient had died, and they went to the hospital. There, with the body, the private nurse, and the wife, the litany for the dying in the 1979 *Book of the Common Prayer* was used. The wife allowed the hospital to use the body for science.

The funeral was "a production," unique, contemporary, and corporate, using media techniques relevant to advertising. The wife took an active, controlled part in the funeral. Her assumption seemed to be that now that P. J. was dead, the pastor's attention would shift to her.

Until her remarriage two years later, the wife used the pastor as a support and resource for her problems. A fellow parishioner assisted her with financial planning. She underwent some depressions and anticipated anniversary reactions by leaving town. One bizarre incident occurred when the hospital called wanting a release for dental records. The lack of a body at the funeral and "to bury" had overtly not been a problem. This tactless call, however, brought to mind that the body was still "somewhere." The wife had put off making a memorial, and this time was chosen to memorialize or figuratively lay her husband to rest.

Perhaps the most important knowledge gained by the pastor, who was one of several in the relatively large, active parish, was that he needed the cooperation of other staff, parishioners, and even his family. For the pastor to devote the time necessary in this case, others were required to share the sense of importance of "helping someone die." Other staff had to be willing to cover for him, support him, and encourage him. The situation also required honesty on the part of the clergyman's family, including the children, to acknowledge that when someone is dying, that takes precedence. Past experience in dealing with his children, with the dying, and with hospitals in general helped a good deal in stepping into this mid-terminal situation as a new pastor.

The ability of a group of parishioners to spend time with the family (wife and son), remember them in prayers, and share their experience with the pastor was positive. At times individuals in this group needed extra help from others; generally, however, they supported one another.

To meet cancer patients at the point of their need and to shift behaviors as their need shifts requires sensitivity and flexibility on the part of the pastor. Pastoral and counseling ideals would not have worked with this patient, and the frustration of getting what *he* wanted from the pastor might have resulted in withdrawal on the part of the patient. The pastor allowed both the family and the circumstances to tell him how he might best help; for a time, at least, it seems that the family drew him in to help them cope with the change going on during the disease progression. Both as a friend and as a pastor, he could relate to this struggling couple and their son.

The pastor was aware of at least some of the cues that the dying give. He allowed the patient to be in control whenever possible. He was sensitive to the compartmentalized roles in which the patient placed people — "a priest was there for the soul." He became a trusted friend, able to "take over the task of the journal" and someone who would "stay" even when things were bad. The cues of the planning of the funeral service were missed, however, possibly because the pastor was caught up in his own denial, his own need to "put off the end," as he "put off" planning the music for the service.

The pastor was available to the family — when they had specific problems he found other professional resources. In addition, parish resources were available through those people who cared for the wife and son while he worked with the patient. He was available in terms of the many hours he spent with the patient, just thinking, and with the wife for counseling. He was available to see the profound rewards in "helping someone die," and he found meaning in his pastoral care.

CHAPTER 2

THE HOSPITAL MILIEU

DIAGNOSIS

THE public in general is cancer conscious. Practical techniques for early diagnosis of symptoms, such as the seven danger signs of cancer, have been well publicized. News media constantly report statistics, human interest stories, and new research developments in the field of cancer cure and care. One patient of my experience correctly diagnosed his leukemia from watching a television show, a medical fiction series that included a discussion of the symptomatology of leukemia.

Cancer patients who may live in fear and isolation with questionable symptoms are finally coerced or incapacitated sufficiently to seek medical advice and assistance. Some patients, with no symptoms, are even more shocked to have the disease process discovered at a routine physical examination.[1] When diagnostic procedures for cancer are beyond the scope of a doctor's office and general laboratory, they are usually done at a local hospital on an in- or outpatient basis.

Unless these diagnostic procedures are clearly positive or negative for cancer, patients may be sent to a larger medical center where more sophisticated and often costly equipment is available. Such a move separates the patient from the support of family, friends, and community; the doctor's referral completes transfer with the impression that something is very wrong, and the patient feels more isolated and helpless if the diagnosis is still unknown.

The testing procedures provide the medical staff with a variety of data for both diagnosis and treatment. The location (s), extent, and kind of tumor (and blood dyscrasias such as leukemia) can usually be determined and evaluated from these

---

[1]Donavon, Marilee and Pierce, Sandra, *Cancer Care Nursing* (New York, Appleton-Century-Crofts, 1976), p. 8.

procedures; surgical procedures are also a part of this evalua-
tion. The results dictate the kind of treatment, the combina-
tions of chemotherapy, surgery, radiation therapy that are
appropriate for a specific cancer.

Individual diagnostic procedures may take several days or
require weeks to reach a conclusion. The procedures are physically exhausting, fraught with human error, frustrating in
length, and expensive. The pastor's focus is support of the
patient and the family during this testing period. Good to
nonexistent communication between the medical staff, patient,
and family places the pastor in a position to facilitate this
process. During this period, previous relationships between the
family and the pastor resulting from their parish life may
change. The stark reality of the cancer crisis has the potential
for deepening real intimacy between family and pastor. On
occasion, however, because cancer patients generally have poor
relationships with others,[2] the pastor may discover he must do
some pastoral assessment and rapport building with the family
and patient.

Perhaps pastoral assessment best takes place initially on an
individual basis during this period. The pastor is available for
support, and to offer hope; however, his main task is to listen
to the various ways in which the family and patient perceive
their present situation. He encourages them to express their
worst fears and to continue communication among family
members of even the "bad news." Good ground work in this
period is important for the future, whatever the diagnosis.

A family will raise many issues that focus on communication
and honesty between family members and the patient — discussion with the patient of such matters as possible diagnosis, and
talking about death; the patient's venting of disassociated anger
on the family; frustration over the diagnostic procedures; and
apparent breeches in the present relationships of family
members. While these issues are raised in an effort to control
the situation and be prepared for any eventuality, the concerns
of the patient and family should not be put off as future im-
probabilities, but explored *now*. It is conceivable that more
opportune times will not arise; discussions of death and dying

[2]LeShan, Lawrence, *You Can Fight for Your Life* (New York, M. Evans and Company,
Inc., 1977), p. 50.

are superfluous when death is actually happening. Families often believe that they are not being told everything by doctors; their suspicions may have a rational foundation, but generally are motivated by anxiety and feelings of helplessness. It is difficult for them to accept that there are unknowns in modern medicine and with cancer.[3]

The size of the medical staff — the attending physicians, the residents, and interns — complicates communication; some have data that is not immediately available to others in the diagnostic process. There is no intent to create tension and ambiguity, yet often one doctor will interpret data to the patient in a way in which another doctor has not. There may also be personal problems on the doctor's part, which stifle communication. Hopefully, medical information is communicated with tact, simplicity, and honesty. Patients have been known to bring medical books to the hospital to translate the plethora of technical information they have received.

The pastor, during the diagnostic period, can suggest that the family and patient ask questions and seek clarification and accurate information. Again, this can only be accomplished if communication channels within the family are open. It is not helpful for the pastor to seek out medical information and control its communication to the family. This merely adds one more process that must be worked through and often complicates the communication. By doing this the pastor will make the family in this circumstance dependent on him, or they will shut him out if he oversteps his role. The patient and family can be encouraged to write down questions and to write down answers. Often, the best method of communication is the one used by one oncologist with his patients. No medical information was given the patient alone. Another family member was always asked to be present for good or bad news. Then, the entire communication within the family could be facilitated and information documented by patient and family member alike. When this method is used, patients will hear what they can cope with and suppress what is not presently important to them. They have the opportunity to check and recheck their facts when they are able to hear them and use these data for

[3]LeShan, *You Can Fight for Your Life*, p. 174.

growth. Moreover, they remain in control of the situation because they have the facts available to function appropriately, control being probably the most important need of the cancer patient.[4]

Control becomes more important as the diagnostic procedures and the hospital milieu begin to dehumanize the person and impinge on privacy, personal habits, and behavior. The "good" patient, by medical standards, who silently acquiesces to all personal treatment, is likely to be the patient who will not fight for life, who will not participate in his own healing, and who responds passively (still in control, it must be noted) to all medical care. The "feisty" patient who appropriately monitors his care and evidences concern for what is happening in the details of hospitalization is more likely to be the patient who will fight for life. This patient is not to be confused, however, with angry, problem patients who spend their hospital stay fighting with staff and physicians alike.[5]

During the diagnostic period, when the patient is not tired and exhausted by numerous procedures, there is an opportunity for the pastor to assess the patient's spiritual resources, to affirm avenues of coping that have been successful in the past, and to suggest referral resources for legitimate concerns that the patient has as a result of the illness and diagnostic process, e.g. financial and family. Continued presence and support through the patient's customary religious practices provide stability and continuity in this transitional, and often changing, period.

The importance of uncovering successful methods of coping with past crises and affirming them with the patient cannot be underestimated. The value of assessing with these patients the positive strengths that are available to them plays an important part in combating their feelings of helplessness, worthlessness, and despair. They do maintain control of how they cope with the situation, and this fact cannot be said enough to them. Prayers, experiences of God's goodness, and sacramental rites can additionally strengthen them as they wait for a final diagnosis.[6]

The diagnosis introduces the element of radical change into

---

[4]Donavon and Pierce, *Cancer Care Nursing*, p. 13.
[5]LeShan, *You Can Fight for Your Life*, p. 43.
[6]LeShan, *You Can Fight for Your Life*, p. 129.

the hospitalization and may alter the patient's life-style and behavior. A pastor cannot assume that two visits on the same day (or even an hour apart) will see the patient in the same circumstances. The ups and downs of the disease process make it difficult and demanding for any helping professional; the situation can change in a five-minute doctor's visit or by a chance comment made during a procedure. The pastor's responsibility in this milieu is to remain with the patient and to be sensitive to whatever new developments arise in the course of the diagnostic process. An effort to apply a standard bandage to the situation results in lessened communication with any patient, particularly so with the cancer patient.

One of the most helpful interventions that the pastor may be able to make during this period for himself, for the family, and for the patient is a clarifying of the meaning of cancer for all involved. What does it mean to possibly have cancer? Public opinion often sees cancer as a death sentence and as an outside force that victimizes those who have the disease.[7] This viewpoint is problematic in the guidance of those who have the disease, and are being treated for it, in their attitudes towards their recovery. Their inability to take responsibility for participating in the disease milieu, and attitude of "being done to," also disassociates them from the participation in being healed. In addition, the belief that the diagnosis of cancer means "death" allows one option to the outcome of the disease process. Cancer, like other diseases, is a chronic illness that is "lived with." To have the attitude that one lives with cancer rather than dies from cancer is to possess an attitude that encourages hope, self-control, and willingness to fight for life. A negative view of the disease process as something one dies with, something terminal, complicates emotional and spiritual care and hinders effective medical treatment.

The meaning of the diagnosis for *each* individual is important. The family and the patient will respond or react in accordance with their perceptions and previous experience of the disease process. Family members who also have cancer or have had it inform the family's responses about the disease process; there is a reality to their comments and consensus that cannot

---

[7]Donavon and Pierce, *Cancer Care Nursing*, p. 3.

be overlooked or ignored. The reality of their information and experience is not the only reality, and their concerns are focused upon aspects of the disease that are particularly horrendous to them. The patient and family are limited in having information about or knowing only a few persons with a few kinds of cancer, rather than having a broad spectrum of data from which to draw their conclusions. Their concerns and worries at this time are normal; continued pastoral presence and supportive counseling with both the patient and family are appropriate during this period.[8]

As the diagnosis comes nearer to being determined, the pastor's task changes. If there is considerable certainty that the tumor is benign, an illness of another kind, tension lessens and the patient and family begin to relax. The emotional buildup that has occurred in the ensuing period of diagnostic procedures begins to dissipate, and when information is finally communicated that malignancy is no longer a concern, the celebration is real and legitimate.

In communication of the diagnosis of cancer, some medical staff insist upon talking to both patient and family, but other medical staff act upon ethical principles that do not recognize the importance of patient and family interaction in illness and health. Either the patient is told the diagnosis and left to choose what and when to tell the family, or the family is told the diagnosis and left to tell or not tell the patient. In either instance, misinformation and dishonesty interfere with interpersonal relationships and the ability to cope with the realities of the disease process.[9] Aside from the likelihood that ensuing treatment cannot otherwise be explained, there are many possibilities that a staff nurse or doctor will let slip the diagnosis or respond to direct questioning from patient or family. The need for family secrets from one another, whatever rationalizations are made, indicates a poorly functioning family. There is also the possibility that the medical situation may alter radically, leaving patient or family angry and confused at the unexpected crisis with which they are now confronted. In addition, the unknown is more frightening to patient or family than the known, fantasies more difficult to deal with than fact, and

---

[8]Donavon and Pierce, *Cancer Care Nursing*, p. 10.
[9]LeShan, *You Can Fight for Your Life*, p. 126.

unexplained feelings more likely to cause pain and suffering.[10]

Case Study

A fifty-two-year-old man had carefully hidden the truth about the seriousness and extent of his illness from his family. He adjusted well to his illness but told his family little about the reoccurrence of his leukemia and hid his rapidly worsening condition. "He always took care of them." He would not allow the doctor to relay any information to them. His wife "wouldn't understand," he said. When he became comatose, and hemorrhaged, the doctor was forced to explain to the angry wife that her husband was critically ill, and that he would soon die. To avoid a lawsuit, he also explained that her husband would not allow him to give her information. Her shock and anger when she discovered the truth made any pastoral care to her and the patient's family impossible while he died. Despite the doctor's ethical explanation that the *husband* was *his* patient, and mentally competent to make such decisions, secrecy created an unreconcilable breech between husband and wife. Perhaps it had always been present in the marriage, yet timely intervention might have prevented some of this situation.

Pastoral authority in a crisis, coupled with a good patient and family rapport, can be used effectively to forestall some of these situations. Although "telling" is often put off because "he" will be upset, the objection generally is more the family's concern for itself. Tears and shock that they wish to avoid are quickly over and are minor incidents compared to the problems created when the illusions left to family or patient are broken. Generally, communication and relationships are improved by openness and honesty.[11]

The communication of the diagnosis of cancer, even though family and patient have, by now, many clues that this might be the case, is a shock, and results in a wide variety of reactions that are generally appropriate to the family patterns of which they are a part. Most are normal reactions; *only* when they are

---

[10]Donavon and Pierce, *Cancer Care Nursing*, p. 9.
[11]Donavon and Pierce, *Cancer Care Nursing*, p. 10.

carried to excess over some period of time do these responses become problematic for the persons involved and for pastoral care.

Talking about the diagnosis is no more an indication of coping with the diagnosis than refusal to discuss it. Disassociation, telling people in detail about the diagnosis and how it was conveyed, without emotion, and reminiscing about what caused the cancer can be as much a denial as silence. Equally problematic is an effort to jump to an anticipated conclusion of death, fantasizing all possible details of the projected future.[12] In an effort to face the reality, to remain in control of the entire situation including the future, patient or family limit themselves to one option of the disease process, be that recovery, denial, or death. The consequences of their behavior and the possibility of other options might be pointed out to them in a tactful manner.

Within a few days the reality of the diagnosis, if commonly known to patient and family, will have penetrated. At this point some feelings, either of sorrow, anger, or despair, may become apparent. These feelings need to be accepted by the pastor, although family members may not be able to listen to the reality of the situation. Generally, even if the patient is not directly told the diagnosis, a number of things happen that convey the message anyway. Tests stop or treatments change, family or long-time friends may "visit," behavior is different among close family members, and even staff responses change. There are innumerable nonverbal clues from which the patient learns his condition. When and if communication about the diagnosis has been open, prospects for treatment generally offer new hope to the situation.

Case Study

Mrs. H. is a seventy-eight-year-old woman, widowed three years, Roman Catholic, and newly admitted for diagnostic tests. She shows evidence of recent weight loss. She tries to be cooperative with the staff and keep up a good appearance physically

---

[12]Donavon and Pierce, *Cancer Care Nursing*, p. 6.

as well as interpersonally. She talks rapidly and frequently. She wanted to be told accurately what would happen to her then have that followed through, becoming irritable when this was not done during her tests. She blurts out on a pastoral visit that her doctor has just told her she has cancer and what treatment she will receive. "It was such a shock." She is telling her family herself. She cries and tries to accept it. She continues talking for about forty-five minutes. The themes for her conversation was typical of newly diagnosed cancer patients.

1. "What did I do wrong?" Mrs. H. confesses that she "used to eat a whole apricot pie on washday" because she was too busy to cook for herself, and it always upset her stomach. (Her cancer is intestinal.) "I didn't know I was harming myself."
2. "I have so much to live for" — her grandchildren are important to her.
3. "Who will take care of me?" — she has taken care of a neighbor for some time, now she needs help.
4. "I hope I will get well" — "My doctors and this hospital helped me get well the last time I was here. It is a good place to be."
5. "Why did this happen to me?" "My sister is eighty-one and so active, and she was always the puny one, but I was big and strong and I was always sick."

Mrs. H. reminisced in the usual way about how she had come to the hospital for diagnosis, noticing her weight loss.

Three days later, Mrs. H. was telling the same story, just beginning to cope with her diagnosis. Although she had talked a great deal in the earlier pastoral visit, she was still in shock, using words she had been told. She did some more crying. Just before her discharge and after her first cobalt treatment, which was begun after four days after her diagnosis, she gave me some religious literature she had been reading. She also had her priest visit for Communion on my suggestion.

Mrs. H.'s comments were typical of patients' concern with their appearance, and their efforts to control the diagnostic situation and their feelings despite shock. Allowing them to talk gives the pastor a good picture of what their experience tells them, e.g. her children may not want to hear the truth, her friends may suspect her disease, she knows she's in shock. Any counseling about these concerns would be done at a later time. She and the family may need help at a later date to make some decisions about who will care for her, bring her to the hospital frequently for cobalt treatments, and where and with whom she will live as she grows weaker.

Her weight loss and her friends' comments as well as the many tests gave her some indication that her disease might be serious. These clues are apparent to every patient and family whether or not they are discussed. Fears of what the future holds both during the testing and thereafter in the course of cancer complicate the patient's comfort. "Living one day at a time" helps keep some control over the fear and counteracts the feelings of helplessness. Typical concerns of how and why this happened, and happened to her, are an effort to find a rational answer to the cause of her sickness. She feels some guilt — did she cause the cancer? She asked these questions of each professional who visited her.

It is easy to mistake open discussion of the doctor's diagnosis as acceptance rather than shock. Confirmation that her discussion of "cancer" was not acceptance came when the pastor observed that Mrs. H. was still in the same shock emotionally after three days.

The situation at the juncture of diagnosis and treatment is a time of many surprises for the patient and the family. They begin to look hesitantly towards the radically changed future of life with cancer. They must make decisions about their treatment based on data that they may not fully understand, or allow their doctor to make these decisions for them. They face additional financial burdens, role changes among family members, and perhaps surgery, with its loss of body image and an alteration of themselves as persons. The effects of treatment, which usually are carefully explained, do not become a reality until they occur; the process of treatment as a whole is with tension, uncertainty, much waiting, and fear of anticipated outcomes.

TREATMENT

Whatever treatment or combination of treatments is selected, there are generally physical side effects. Because the patient must sign documents attesting to an understanding of the doctor's explanation of these treatments, the entire process is usually well explained and appears to be understood at the time. However, the amount of medical terminology used in the explanation, a continuing need for denial, and difficulty in understanding the implications of what has been said often result in the patient's assessment that the doctor was not clear in communicating what side effects occur as a result of treatment. Even when confronted with the question, "Didn't the doctor tell you this?", and an affirmative response, it is clear that the patient did not really *expect* whatever is happening to him. There appears to be a difference between what was understood and what actually happened.

In addition, adjustments must be made during treatment for individual patient responses to chemo- or radiation therapy, and these situations are often not predictable by medical staff. To patient and family who hoped that *this* treatment would be "the answer" to illness and bring a cure, the frustration of these adjustments accompanied by the other radical changes that the disease forces upon them cause fear, anger, and despair. The pastoral goal in this treatment period is helping the family and patient to cope with the effects that treatment has upon the physical and emotional behavior of the patient, to support them whatever happens, lessening their anxiety, and using their resources to help them through.

Although the side effects of chemotherapy and radiation treatments are clearly described as nausea, hair loss, etc., most patients deny that the side effects are happening or will happen to them. Despite the beginning of hair loss, when a woman patient said that her hair "was coming out in clumps on the pillow," she followed this statement by saying that she "didn't think that that side effect would happen" to her. Nausea is most often experienced as food tasting bad, although that can be a separate side effect. The accompanying fatigue, sleepiness, and irritability are bewildering to the family and friends. Visitors are tolerated, but disturb the patient's rest. Those patients who need to keep up a "good appearance" to everyone are most uncomfortable if this becomes difficult or impossible. They may be angry and withdraw when the effort to "feel fine" becomes too great. Pastoral visits, based on the patient's present condition and wishes, are important, allowing the patient to be in control of the visit; being willing to be quietly with the patient, not talking much; and respecting the patient's need even to be left alone. Short, warm visits without any expectations of a visit at all are appropriate goals. There are occasions when, if the pastor has shown himself to be available, the patient may wish to talk, but it repeatedly must be stressed that the patient's needs come first. The drug side effects add to the sense of illness and helplessness that the patient already feels and may result in some unusual behavior. If the pastoral relationship is to be effective, these new dimensions of the disease must be respected.

Continued side effects result in a loss of morale. It is difficult for patients and families to understand how the increased symptoms caused by the therapies can help healing, and the results are often frightening to all. To a woman who is proud of her appearance, hair loss can be devastating. The reactions of her friends to her altered appearance move her closer to despair. A man who is unable to eat any food or who has sores caused by the lowered body resistance during therapy often feels loss of control of his illness and his masculine image. Other consequences occur on an individual basis to patients who do not wish family and friends, and even spouses, "to see me like this." It may be possible to relay these concerns to the nursing staff as the pastor becomes aware of them. Education by those trained to help cope with these changes and by volunteers trained to talk to patients who have problems such as they have had are often available and helpful.

Case Study

Mr. L. was a fifty-one-year-old man who was married and has two adopted daughters. He was Lutheran. He had been hospitalized for seven weeks with the diagnosis of leukemia, for which he received IV chemotherapy. He had two courses of the chemotherapy with about two weeks between them because of infections and sores on his mouth, which were painful, disfiguring, and interfered with his eating. Although he did not appear to listen to the education regarding chemotherapy that his nurse gave him, he showed what she wrote down to other visitors, including the pastor.

Early in the treatment process, he was intensely agitated, in constant motion on and off the bed, moving about his room. He talked about going home soon so that he could go on his regular fishing vacation with friends. He could only discuss his illness and treatment as "needing to know what was going on." He expressed no feelings about having cancer or more chemotherapy. His wife visited frequently, bringing food, which they offered to visitors as he could not eat it. She seemed pleasant, controlled, calm, and with little emotional expression.

When he felt well, he made paintings and other handicrafts, which he enjoyed showing to visitors. What he did seemed to give him a sense of worth. While ill from the chemotherapy, he slept a great deal and finally lay quietly in his bed, a great contrast from his earlier behavior. At the end of the second course of treatment, while waiting for the test results, he admitted to feeling discouraged. He talked about "patient's rights" and "doctors not telling the patients everything." He was told that he might have to have a third or fourth round of chemotherapy, and he felt that "they should have told me this at the beginning." He would not further express his feelings about the possibility of more chemotherapy, however, but lay in bed staring at the blank TV set. He appeared to be increasingly depressed. Since his lip had healed, he was allowed to go home on a pass for the weekend.

When he returned from the pass, his tests were clear and he came bouncing up to several medical staff in the hall to celebrate. He returned to the hospital six weeks later for another checkup. All was well with him; his leukemia was in remission.

Mr. L. appeared to be in constant motion to compensate for his feelings of helplessness. He needed to be "doing," and "giving" constantly. He had difficulty expressing his feelings about his illness to any staff members, but was able to ask for help and discuss other matters of concern to him. His pastor visited about once a week, and Mr. L. and his wife appeared grateful for the pastor's concern.

The issue of "not being told everything" probably would not have occurred if Mr. L. had had one treatment and then gone home. The additional chemotherapy and treatment of the lip ulcers delayed his recovery for several weeks. This could not be foreseen, and this man had hopes and expectations of discharge within three weeks. When his hospitalization dragged on for more than a month and the chemotherapy had to be repeated, he had additional concerns, not only his illness, but of what would happen to his job, his plans, his wife and children. The cost of hospitalization and treatment left this man with an estimated bill of about $10,000 for seven weeks of treatment. However, it also left him with an indefinite time to live a relatively normal life.

Responses to therapy do become critical in some cases, and a process designed to heal may fail. Good medical management should prevent this in most instances, and support and encouragement keep the patient fighting, but this does not happen in all instances. The treatment process, with its effects and tedious procedures, results in depression, accompanying the feelings of helplessness and the loss of control that the patient is experiencing and may be unable to express. Even though the patient is encouraged to ventilate these feelings, earlier emotional patterns make release of these feelings difficult, and the family response may be such that these feelings cannot be talked about.

Intervention to allow the patient to be as much in control of his care as possible includes having the patient make decisions about small matters with which he or she can cope, such as how the room will be arranged, door open or closed, and menu choice. It may be possible for the pastor to suggest this to the family. However, there are family patterns in which the family's need to control the situation and the patient is greater than the patient's, and although the family should assist in care when possible, some patterns of behavior are not helpful to anyone. A family member who remains with the patient day and night, heedless of personal care and neglectful of other responsibilities, generally has a burden of guilt and dependency feelings towards the patient, which are being acted out. The pastor encourages these family members to take care of themselves so that they can be available to the patient. Equally suspect is the family that never shows up when they can visit, virtually abandoning the patient to nursing care. In such pastoral matters as sacramental actions, the pastor who has not been available may now be requested not to come, for the patient "might think he is going to die," and again, the family's need to control the situation prevents the patient from making his needs known. The alternative response to the pastor may be a demand by the family for constant attention and daily visits. It appears that the family members look to the pastor to relieve some of their burden. they may also have needs for more pastoral care than they can ask for themselves.

Chemotherapy and radiation treatment that can be done on an outpatient rather than an inpatient hospital basis are preferable, since the return to daily routine at home tends to be a morale booster. The patient who lives alone needs to be regularly in communication with a caring person so that if chemotherapy creates side effects, a situation in which the patient cannot care for himself, someone is available to help.

After the beginning of treatment, the pastor will at times be confronted with the question of cessation of treatment. He will likely hear the family raise the issue in an ambivalent manner as they discuss the treatment of disease process. Particularly if there is a reoccurrence of the tumor or if other family members have had cancer, families will express a wish "not to see him suffer." Usually, the pastor can pick up on these statements and open them for discussion. Generally, although the patient and the family members talk among themselves, unless the situation has been long drawn out and severe, they will not say the same things to the doctor. Attitudes of the medical staff are changing towards ethical issues of these kinds, and certainly the doctor who is aware of these comments will check with the family members from time to time to see if their wishes have changed. It can be helpful for the pastor to facilitate this communication; it is inappropriate for him to make such decisions for or with the family, or to relate to medical staff in the place of family members even when seeking additional information about the patient. Interference in the family coping mechanisms can result in a rupture in the relationship between pastor and family or an overly dependent family, rendering them increasingly unable to rely upon their own resources.

Treatment that involves surgical procedures causes more immediate short-term tension. These procedures may include diagnostic surgery, therapeutic surgery, and palliative surgery; the patient's and the family's response to surgery depends upon the unknowns present when the surgery was undertaken. The results of surgery may be a detailing of the extent of the spread of the disease and that the problem is cancer, that the entire tumor was removed, or that the surgeon did what was possible to insure more time for life and relative comfort. Surgery may be followed by chemotherapy or radiation treatments as a precautionary measure against possible reoccurrence. There are several organizations that are staffed by trained volunteers who educate and support patients coping with postoperative problems such as ostomies and mastectomies.[13]. Some medical staff will not permit these volunteers to visit their patients while hospitalized. Referrals must be made by the doctor.

Completion of the therapy treatments generally result in improved physical and emotional condition. There are additional tests to assess the effectiveness of the treatment. Waiting for these test results is generally a tense time. If the remission or regression of the cancer is incomplete, additional chemotherapy or radiation treatments will be used; the cycle of treatment begins again. If the results are good, the patient will go home with follow-ups by his doctor, and the resumption of "normal" life begins. There is the continued concern that the disease will reoccur. This fear needs to be ventilated when possible and acknowledged as a potential reality. Reoccurrence is possible; nevertheless, fear should not so preoccupy the patient and family that their life becomes untenable.[14] Should this occur,

---

[13]American Cancer Society, *Free Help*, pamphlet, Chicago, 1976.
[14]Simonton, Carl and Simonton, Stephanie, "Belief systems and Management of the Emotional Aspects of Malignancy," *Journal of Transpersonal Psychology*, 7:36, 1975.

therapy or counseling is recommended to help them deal with this concern. Although this fear is repressed by other patients, any physical symptoms become a cause for special concern, and some of this concern is healthy, motivating the patient to have these symptoms checked by the doctor.

RECURRENCE

The recurrence of cancer necessitates the reworking of the acceptance process, almost as though there were a new disease present. If the patient and family had assumed that the remission, therapy, or surgery meant that they would no longer be bothered by cancer, they will be angry, discouraged, and disappointed. Denial of the recurrence will likely not be prolonged if communication is clear about diagnosis. Helplessness and depression are more prevalent; the hope that the last treatment would work is gone. The patient is more likely to be thinking about death and, more importantly, about how he wants to live the time left. The focus of pastoral conversations may be on the quality rather than the quantity of life. The patient and family have differing views on how this occurs, and their views may be irreconcilable. In addition, the doctors and medical staff wish to try other treatments, some of which will be experimental, and so the conflict shifts not to death itself, but how that will happen for this patient. The patient knows exactly what will happen during treatment and can realistically assess the suffering and discomfort he will experience. This time gained by treatment is evaluated against the days and months spent in treatment. If the recurrence is within months or a year of the original illness, the patient may even be more reluctant to try new treatment, while persons who have gained four or five years are more likely to see treatment as the opportunity for "more time."[15]

Case Study

A thirty-eight-year-old, single woman, Miss R., Roman Cath-

---

[15]Donavon and Pierce, *Cancer Care Nursing*, p.26.

olic, has a recurrence of cancer of the breast with metastases to several areas of the body. She lives with her parents and works as a secretary and a waitress. Her recurrence was discovered in a medical checkup after two years of being disease free. She had a mastectomy and chemotherapy for her previous disease.

On the pastor's first visit Miss R. says how much she appreciates the doctor's directness in telling her of the recurrence. She "had a feeling" this might be the case. She believes that the recurrence is "God's will" for her, but she wants prayer for "a miracle." Although she was told about the recurrence, she moves restlessly about the room. Her religious life is such that she wants a pastor present and Holy Communion.

Later, while she is still having medical tests to determine the extent of the disease and possible treatment, she talks for a long time about options that face her. She talks about wanting "to die with dignity." She's been through this before, and she is not sure she wants more treatment. Miss R. explored this in depth, examining her life's goals. Was there anything she wanted to do with the rest of her life? She wanted to "do something," for her parents, and felt she had an "obligation" to them. She believes in miracles and wants to take her parents "on a trip to Lourdes." She said that when her parents found out about her recurrence, her father "prayed up a storm, and when he prays, things happen." He had come to visit that night saying, "We have just begun to fight." However, she had every confidence in her doctor's decisions. The doctor had planned removal of her ovaries to decrease hormone production, and thereby hopefully affect the tumor. The patient complied with this treatment.

Postsurgically, there was no more talk about her dying. There were many complaints about poor nursing care, similar to her complaint in her earlier hospitalization. The nurses did not bring pain medications, did not give her good care. Moreover, she did not like more doctors looking at her body. She was dischared two weeks later and the nursing staff was relieved to see her go, as her parents had also been complaining. Several months later, a note said she was back at work.

Miss R. maintained much control over her appearance and her situation. She was ambivalent about the reoccurrence of her disease, but had carefully considered the alternative of death with dignity. Although she talked about it freely and needed to do this, by the end of the conversation, when she had taken her parents' and the doctor's wishes into account (and perhaps her own wishes were projected upon them), she was willing to abide by the doctor's decisions for treatment. Her anger at the situation took the form of irritability at the nursing staff.

At times Miss R. appeared to be very calm and independent, but her behavior with the doctor and her parents seemed very dependent. Her religious ideation seemed immature in some senses, both her wishes for miracles and her belief that what had happened to her was "God's will." Although she discussed these issues to some degree with the pastor and made frequent use of the sacraments of her church, she did not seem to move much from this stance, and talked very little about religion after her surgery.

There are times, too, when the doctor frankly admits there is nothing more he or the medical profession have to offer for treatment. The response to this statement is often relief, a renewed desire to fight on, resignation, or hopelessness. Physical condition may be so poor at this point that another issue is raised, and that is one of care outside the hospital. The family situation may be such that care at home is impossible, or if it is available as the cancer progresses, it becomes untenable later on. Whenever this occurs, even in other illness, the decision to place the patient in an extended care facility or nursing home is an extremely difficult one for family and patient alike.

The feelings of guilt that the family has are the primary pastoral problem.[16] Family members may not wish to tell the patient that a stay in the nursing home is what will happen to him or her, and they may construct stories about the patient staying in the care facility until he or she is stronger, or refuse to use the name "nursing home." Usually they must deal with the arrangements they make. However, the patient, too, will need help to express the angry feeling he or she may have

---

[16]Donavon and Pierce, *Cancer Care Nursing*, p. 35.

towards the family and towards the illness for causing this situation. Occasionally, this solution to the home care program can cause bizarre behavior in an already ill patient. If there is a possibility of the family discussing these arrangements with the patient, there is also the possibility that the patient will understand. One of the primary concerns of the cancer patient is that he or she does not wish to be a burden upon the family as the illness progresses. However, the patient and the family may have different views as to what the realities of home care involve. This, too, creates problems for all involved. Visiting nurses and social workers can help to provide an objective assessment of what the family and patient can expect from one another. The emotional problems and conflicts created by a cancer patient with the ups and downs of the daily care of the patient are often as exasperating and difficult for the family to cope with and understand as are the physical aspects of patient care. Hopefully, resource persons will be available who can discuss some of these problems with the family throughout the remaining process of the illness.

CHAPTER 3

CANCER — THE "TERMINAL" ILLNESS

FROM CHRONIC TO CRITICAL

IN a real sense we are all terminal; we all die.
Cancer is a chronic disease rather than terminal illness per se.
The attitudes that stress "living with cancer" and a positive
outlook for treatment and recovery, or at least stability in treatment, are important for the healing process of the cancer patient. These attitudes are difficult to maintain because of the
psychological patterns of the cancer patient. Often the family
stresses one aspect or the other of the illness, optimism or
despair.[17] The ups and downs of the disease, the day-to-day
changes from good to poor physical condition, are precisely
those aspects of the disease which make cancer so problematic
as a pastoral situation. There is a real tension between living
with hope for recovery and denial of the reality of this chronic
illness; one or the other predominates in the family or patient
responses to cancer. Generally, the appropriate pastoral stance
is to support the patients in their struggle to cope with the
present, accepting their feelings for today and allowing both
patient and family to maintain the defenses they need. It is
probably best to leave these defenses unchallenged until or
unless they seriously interfere with total care of the family. The
patients summarize feelings about the terminal part of their
disease when they say, "when I feel bad, I want to die and when
I feel good, I want to live." After a prolonged illness the family
may have similar feelings, taking hope on the good days and
despairing on the bad days.

At some undefined point in this chronic illness, the cancer
patient begins to let go of life. This point is determined by the
patient's physical condition, age, length of illness, emotional

---

[17]LeShan, *You Can Fight for Your Life*, p. 174.

state, and other factors. Few doctors nowadays will be pushed into predicting life expectancy for any kind of cancer at the beginning of the illness, and fewer still at the end of the illness. Perhaps at the very end they may predict a day or an hour, but they are often outdone by a tenacious patient who clings on past all understanding, or stymied by a patient who dies almost without warning.[18]

Although the patient and usually the family are concerned about pain and suffering, as a rule there is little, the patient sliding off into sleep and then death. Modern medication alleviates most pain. There are occasionally very difficult and problematic deaths when the tumor process has affected brain or lungs, or in some of the blood diseases. Pastoral presence can be helpful as long as it is quiet and supportive. This process may take days or weeks, or sometimes the patient will show a remarkable, short recovery. The family may take hope at this time, but generally it is not realistic response to what is happening. Nursing staff may also be responding to the death by either denial or despair, and it can be important for the pastor to trust his own views about what is happening to the patient and family *if* the pastor has worked through his own emotional problems with death.[19] Generally, the patient and family have had some time to adjust to approaching death.

Adjustment manifests itself consistently in the behavior patterns of the patient and family. For example, those patients who are accustomed to being in control of their lives are not likely to lose control of their situation now. Familiar coping mechanisms used in excess by both the patient and the family become inappropriate and sometimes alienate others involved in their care, including the pastor. It is important to insist on responsible and mature behavior on the part of the patient and family. Babying a patient or allowing the family to behave inappropriately because of a critical situation is not helpful to them or to the hospital.[20]

Among the problem behaviors is a syndrome best described

---

[18]Kubler-Ross, Elizabeth, *On Death and Dying* (New York, The Macmillan Company, 1969), p. 99.

[19]Kubler-Ross, *On Death and Dying*, p. 227.

[20]LeShan, *You Can Fight for Your Life*, p. 172.

as the "do something" syndrome. It has many facades, but it is generally manifested in the patient's increased demands that the family and nursing staff "do something" for the patient. The underlying wish is that someone, anyone, will "do something" about the patient's critically ill status, to hold back the threat of death and the feelings of loss of control that panic the patient. Occasionally, frustrated family members will make similar demands resulting from the helplessness they feel. Generally, patient and family are also angry, and this communicates itself to the staff, who become equally angry at the constant demands and requests that manipulate them. Nursing staff in particular struggle to cope with the stream of requests, making care plans to guide them in helping the patient maintain as much personal control as possible while countering the dependency that these demands create. Some staff members who are unable to cope with the patients withdraw as the patient's behavior becomes more manipulative and excessive.[21]

Helping the patient to face feelings of helplessness is a problem of utmost tact. Patients need to be helped to "do something" for themselves as often as possible. If they have been active people, the limitations of an illness alone sufficiently frustrate them. Breaking down the simplest acts into manageable components by all those caring for the patient, including the pastor (who is also likely to be drawn into these demands), indicates to the patient that others believe he or she is in control and has some coping skills. For example, in responding to a request to call the nurse: "Here is your call button. I'll put it in your hand. Now you can press the button when you want to," or "How would you like your door, open or closed?" This kind of decision making is vital to the well-being of the patient and is an action in which all who participate convey respect and interest to the patient. Requests for prayer and sacraments can be handled in the same way by asking what the patient wants to pray for or what Scripture he wants read, rather than handing out a "tried-and-true" format.[22]

Some allusions to dying are generally made during this time. The family may not wish to hear the patient say, "I've about

---

[21]Kubler-Ross, *On Death and Dying*, p. 45.
[22]Kubler-Ross, *On Death and Dying*, p. 48.

had it," or "I'm ready to go." Allowing the patient to discuss these feelings can be important to his or her well-being. The dying process is such that the family and the patient may not be at the same place in the process, one more accepting of the event than others. Probing for such disclosure on the pastor's part suggests that the need to talk about death is more his than the patient's if there has been no cue from the patient.

Patient concern for family members "after I die" and how to tell them what is happening is normal. The family makes the assumption in most cases that the person who is dying does not know it. The absurdity of this event happening unknown to anyone who is terminally ill reflects a *wish* rather than fact. When the patient does try to tell the family members what is happening, they either deny it or are surprised by it. Patients struggling to remain in control may go so far as to detail who the surviving spouse is to remarry. These comments must be treated with seriousness, and not misunderstood or ignored.[23]

DEATH AND THE DYING

"Abide with me, fast falls the even tide" — an old hymn sums up the ministry to the terminally ill. Generally, the dying patient does not want to be alone. He may convey this wish in various ways. One patient in the author's experience had the television on and the lights on and the door open, clinging to the last stimuli of life as she died. Other patients close the door and muffle and darken the room, and all speak in hushed tones. Only rarely will a patient ask everyone to leave when he or she senses that death has come.

Most families will conduct bedside vigils, which are appropriate as long as the family cares for itself, too. The family has the opportunity to come to grips with reality, to say what it needs to say and do what it needs to do to prepare itself for the impending loss. Being with a terminally ill patient, however long the final illness lasts, can be a rewarding and fulfilling task for all. It is a time to see life in all its reality, to learn about courage and love from those who are about to die. Physical and

---

[23]Kubler-Ross, *On Death and Dying*, p. 101.

mental deterioration can cloud this time, however, and further pastoral care to either patient or family may be determined by the progress of this deterioration. Hopefully, physical and mental processes deteriorate simultaneously, for this lessens the problems that face the family in this proccess.

Physical deterioration, when the patient is aware of the increase in physical helplessness and loss of bodily functions, is painful for all. Efforts to continue communication between patient and family require creative ideas such as a sign or picture boards and a great deal of patience. Often the patient may communicate by writing notes when speech is no longer possible. If previous pastoral care has been appropriate, support at this time, through presence and touch, is meaningful; the effort to talk is too great to "make conversation." If the pastor evidences discomfort and an inability to cope with the dying, he will not be used as a resource by the family.

Mental deterioration is more problematic and frightening to the family. They are bewildered by delusions, angry responses, and an inapproprate behavior. They do not know what to make of the changes in the family member and often wonder if this side of the patient was one they suspected might be present. Patient's comments generally include enough of reality to make them plausible, as though they are long-suppressed material now coming into the open. In the same way, attitudes about family members appear to surface that have been "held in" for years. The family may respond with guilt or anger to these comments, trying to keep the patient quiet even by means of drugs. Occasionally, issues of sexuality or even comments of frank psychosis are made; then just as suddenly, the patient may become lucid again for unpredicatable lengths of time. In addition, responses to medication may produce similar emotional outbursts.

There are many indications that a comatose patient can hear and is aware of what is being said about him or to him in the room. This observation may be used helpfully or harmfully in this terminal stage when patients often drift in and out of coma. It is not helpful for the family to discuss the patient's condition as though he were not present or to say things that would not be said if he were alert. This behavior merely dehumanizes the patient and further disturbs the relationships between the family and patient.

Touching and talking to the patient, saying those things that the family needs to say, should be encouraged, so that there is no unfinished business. In addition, some families use this time to summarize and eulogize all that the patient's life has been, reminiscing among themselves. In this way they reassure the patient that he is not alone, and that life has been of value and their relationships have had meaning. There is time for reconciliation. Indeed, it sometimes appears that a patient will not die until some relative or friend from the past has come. Whatever the need, and it may never be clear, there appears to be some purpose served by that particular visit from a person who has lived at a physical or psychological distance.

There are families who have celebrations in the patient's room — a birthday, a wedding — and these draw the patient into the life of the family. Any liturgical service, etc., which is significant to the family, may be modified so that the cancer patient can share in one more family event.

On occasion, the family, in an effort to hold off the encroachment of death, is reluctant to invite family members from out of town to pay a final visit. The pastor is in a position to encourage the family to notify these members of the situation and give them an opportunity for reconciliation. Pastoral authority used here by an objective onlooker can be a way of facilitating the family's decisions around the final crisis. Generally, the family is not as functional as it might ordinarily be. However, too much intervention will be rejected. Again, sensitive use of sacrament and prayer will be helpful to support the family and to summarize the events of the past and present and the hope of the future.

Family response to death depends upon the length of time the family has had to cope with the probability of the event, and the *real* intimacy of the relationships. There is a need both to be present at the time of death and a wish not to be present, a desire to support the dying person and continue the relationship to the end, and a fear of the encounter with finitude and mortality. When the patient dies, the focus for pastoral care shifts to the family members for their lives go on, forever altered by their loss. They continue to need pastoral support, and the funeral service can be a summary and a finalizing of the loss event. Yet, the gap left by the patient's death remains, and mourning continues for many months after the moss.[24] Emotional support by the pastor in this period is an important part of the healthy working through their loss. Many studies have shown that disease processes that include cancer follow the death of loved ones. Pastoral presence and counseling in these situations is active intervention focused upon the loss events that appear to trigger or initiate these processes.

[24]Marris, Peter, *Loss and Change* (New York, Pantheon Books, 1974), p. 35.

CHAPTER 4

PASTORAL CARE AND COUNSELING

MODERN medical complexities often leave parish pastors bewildered by the hospital milieu. Medical developments, terminology, machinery and procedures, referral resources, and specialized medical staff are threatening and overwhelming in the sheer size and the skill of their offerings. The objectivity created by machinery and evaluative tests adds to the depersonalization of a patient's hospital experience. Here, it seems, into impersonal relationships that often characterize the hospital admission and treatment program, the pastor brings elements of identity and community that can support and sustain the hospital patient.[25]

The Christian community knows a patient as a person and family member. The parish has shared the patient's religious life, history, and growth, and ideally has been the recipient of a patient's gifts. A pastor's presence in crisis is an assurance of the patient's membership in the community and an affirmation of his value and worth. The pastor and members of the congregation are reminders of God's love and care for each individual.

Pastors who minister to cancer patients and their families find a fulfilling and rewarding experience. They learn lessons of courage and love; they wonder at the nature of disease and sin in human lives. The pastor is privileged to listen and to share with cancer patients their journey through "the valley of the shadow of death" as a guide, a shepherd, and a companion. In this pastoral relationship, the pastor must be aware of personal feelings about the many crises that occur in the journey of the cancer patient. Role changes, bodily dysfunction, financial problems, and death, as well as ethical issues, are raised in

---

[25] Jernigan, Rev. Homer L., "Bringing Together Psychology and Theology, Reflections on Ministry to the Bereaved," *Journal of Pastoral Care, 30 (2)*:98, 1976.

the disease process of cancer. Questions concerning the value and meaning of life, as well as profound theological problems, are posed many times during the course of diagnosis and treatment. These issues are of importance to the patient and family as well as germane to the nature of pastoral intervention, requiring therefore, the necessity of the pastor's personal reflection upon them in some way prior to the crisis itself.

There are, however, few clear-cut issues in the ministry to cancer patients. The rapid changes, the multitude of unknown factors in medical and spiritual healing, and even the cultural response to the disease complicate pastoral care. Perhaps the most important asset a pastor to cancer patients may have is the ability to remain flexible and to feel comfortable without being in control of a situation amidst the efforts of others to control, to predict, and to structure the entire hospitalization. The acceptance with which the pastor views his own feelings of helplessness and fear and with which he encounters hopelessness is that dimension of faith which the pastor models for others, sustaining them in spite of the crisis of cancer. It is difficult to share and see the misery that the cancer patients and the family experience without being angry at "someone" for allowing "something" like cancer to happen to people. It is still more difficult to understand how people respond to stress and their life situations in such a way that they become vulnerable to this disease, how they can participate in this illness, and why some get well and some die. We as pastors listen and wait and hope; we know with surety that God is able to redeem and heal. At times when our surety is shaken, when we are caught up with the same hopelessness and helplessness of the family and friends, we too are confronted with the mystery of life and death and God. Then it is time to care for ourselves, to take a day off to pray, to renew our courage, and find strength in ourselves. By surrounding ourselves for a time with the things of living, we return able to continue our sharing of the crisis of cancer.

As pastors we need to remain as objective as possible about our pastoral care to our patients. This is particularly important if we have more than one critically ill patient or family in our parish or institution. Identification with the family or the patient makes it more difficult for us to be sensitive to their needs. The pastor will be involved in the crisis in a way that may interfere with healthy functioning. Attitudes of trust, love, and acceptance towards the cancer patient and family members affirm their own strength in dealing with the crisis. Affirmation for the steps they make in coping, helping to explore past successful methods of dealing with crisis, and affirmation for their openness and willingness to share are ways in which the pastor can continue to model and assist the patient and the family in change. It is not realistic for the pastor to expect them to spend most of their time discussing "serious" issues. They, too, need to put aside the realities of the situation for a time. They need the assurance that normal things are happening, that life is going on, that their lives are going on. The family and the patient will be drawn again and again into confrontation with the disease and the crisis of faith that cancer brings. There is little way to avoid it altogether, and they need all the supportive and caring dimensions that the pastor can bring to bear in this crisis situation. To accomplish these pastoral goals, the pastor may find it imperative to examine and deepen his spiritual life as an outcome of his ministry to cancer patients.[26] The pastor, too, makes a spiritual journey.

SYMBOLIC LANGUAGE

In the process of listening to the cancer patient, and listening is probably the most important part of this ministry, the pastor will hear, with a "third" ear so to speak, a great deal of symbolism language. Most philosophies that discuss symbolism see the symbol as language that objectifies an experience and perceives common elements in an experience of reality.[27] For cancer patients, use of symbolic language takes place when they are unable to talk directly about the reality (usually death) that confronts them. They are simply too frightened to verbalize their feelings or even the word *death* in any other way. Their language is reality oriented and, like dreams, the symbols may

[26]Jerniran, "Bringing Together," p. 98.
[27]Whitehead, Alfred, *Symbolism, Its Meaning and Effect* (New York, The Macmillan Co.,) 1927, p. 8.

be interpreted or raised up into consciousness so that their fears and feelings can be shared.[28] Symbolic language may be used in the context of short phrases, one or two words, themes, and short stories. It may express fears or facts and may be accompanied by nonverbal data. Bringing the symbolic issues and themes open into dialogue must be handled with care. They are a defense that the patient needs to maintain as long as he perceives it necessary.

Perhaps the most common language symbol used by cancer patients, and also many dying patients, is "going home." If this symbol points to a reality, e.g. the patient *is* going home, there will also be references to a specific place or time. The medical staff will say that discharge — "going home" — is to take place. If, however, "going home" is preferred as a chance remark, when there is every indication that the patient is not to be discharged, it often happens that the patient dies in the near future.

Words and short phrases often are unique to the person or the culture. Examples of these might be "having my bags packed," "hanging up my shoes," "wanting to get out" (usually of bed). All kinds of phrases are accompanied by appropriate feelings of hopelessness and helplessness. The words and phrases generally are used in the context of the critical situation but appear inappropriate to the surface level of reality, e.g. the patient is too weak to get out of bed, or the bags are empty suitcases on the floor. The family is generally too invested and too conflicted to help the grief process and to hear the patient's cues. Occasionally, however, they may respond appropriately to the patient's symbolic language on a preconscious level.

Case Study

A seventy-eight-year-old woman in good health lived in an extended care facility. In the fall, in response to a routine visit from her pastor, she looked out the window and said, "What will happen to those flowers when winter comes?" The pastor responded that since they had bulbs, they would come back in

---

[28] Jernigan, "Bringing Together," p. 97.

the spring. The woman began to reminisce about the loss of her husband and the breakup of her home. Then she asked about her cat. Did her cat have a good home? Her pastor responded that she was sure the cat had found a good home. The depression of the patient and the seeming morbidness of the conversation, which focused on dying and loss, prompted the pastor to ask if the woman was ill. She was in good health and the staff did not expect her to die. However, in the winter she died suddenly. Her symbolic language seemed to focus on death and her concerns for care — and life after death.

Typical of nonverbal cues are times in which the patient drifts off into sleep during a conversation, perhaps in preparation for a final sleep. The inability to sleep itself is often based upon the patient's fear of loss of control: if he falls asleep he might not reawaken at all — he will die. Additional nonverbal cues could be a patient's holding on tightly to a sheet or bed rail as holding on to life, dying flowers in the room, or wanting the door left open (to light and life) or closed tightly (a finish, a closure to the world).

Case Study

A sixty-year-old woman hospitalized with cancer of the liver for several months had complications from her chemotherapy. Weakened, she struggled to get well. The possibility of more procedures and more chemotherapy angered and depressed her. As she talked about the futility of more procedures, she pushed a straw up and let it snap down saying, "I just get up and they push me down." She picked up the straw and shoved it in a book, leaving only a little bit sticking out. She died two weeks later. For her, the additional procedures were "the last straw" and she did indeed have only a little (time) left.

The listener must be objective about the patient and the crisis situation so as to discern the symbols that convey the patient's message. The most effective way of surfacing such a message would be to suggest the possible feeling or theme and encourage verbalization of the reality when it accompanies it. The patient may not or cannot discuss these crisis issues; nevertheless, they should be made aware of the continued availability of the pastor, who listens and shares the crisis with them. In one sense, the symbolic language itself is one special way of binding men together by the common emotions that it elicits, particularly the common reality of human death.[29]

People may identify with objects that have special meaning to them. The symbol synthesizes the experience of reality, the person, and the perceived event. The *why* of this relationship need not be understood, for it is the meaning that is important.

Case Study

A sixty-two-year-old woman with cancer of the liver and colon took her father's billy club from beside the bed. She described how the newsboy had been bothering her by tapping on her window at night. He has been "coming to collect what she owed him." She had the club there to fight him off. As she talked she put the club in her other hand and dropped it behind the bed. She died two weeks later. It would appear that death was the newsboy she was fighting, and that she had given up the fight.

These stories are often part of the talk of normally lucid patients and may sometimes be dismissed as psychotic ramblings. However, although symbolic associations are preconscious and individualistic, there are exceptions. A particularly striking example was apparent to the entire nursing staff.

Case Study

A seventy-year-old woman with metastatic cancer had been given a votive (worship) candle by her pastor. It became clear that she believed that when the candle went out she would die. Three days later when the candle burned out she had not died. She remarked to one of the nurses that she guessed she could not order her own death (although it was obvious that she had

---

[29]Whitehead, *Symbolism*, p. 68.

hoped to do so). Her identification with the candle, her burning out or being extinguished, was clear and unusually open.

Sensitivity to these meanings may require nothing further of the pastor. His comments would likely be met by denial from patient and family. Understanding the dynamics of the symbolic language, however, gives the pastor an opportunity to work more closely with the family in preparation for the eventuality of death. He at least "has gotten the message."

PRAYER AND RITES OF PASSAGE

The pastor who uses prayer as a substitute for interpersonal relationships and a jovial cheerup as a contradictory indication of the serious ministry to the cancer patient will lose the depth of that ministry to both the cancer patients and their families. He becomes no more than a superficial visitor to the bedside. This is not to suggest that prayer and sacraments are inappropriate in any way, but merely that they are a means of ministry and not an end.[30]

It is unfortunate, too, that requests for prayer are often couched in terms of prayer *for* a patient rather than praying with a patient. For cancer patients, this mode of request interferes with their opportunity to establish and continue their relationship with God and affirm their self-worth by offering their own petitions. In addition, their request for the pastor to "do something" is a part of their response to the feelings of helplessness caused by their disease. Most patients would benefit from having a short prayer that they might say on their own, and most do have something of this sort among their spiritual resources if they are reminded of this.

Prayer is especially effective not only as part of the healing process but also as a therapeutic summary of the issues of the pastoral visit, an amplification of the pastoral needs. Using this opportunity also to explore the needs in the context of the request may also be a singular opportunity during the pastoral

[30]Carlozzi, Carl G. *Death and the Contemporary Man* (Grand Rapids, Michigan, William B. Erdmans Publishing Co., 1968), p. 56.

visit and an opening for a more intimate discussion of the cancer crisis. Requests for prayer may be made for the pastor for many reasons, some helpful to the patient and some not, but they must be responded to with respect and individuality. Otherwise, the depersonalization of the patient continues in the hospitalization.

In this aspect, prayers that are found in devotional manuals for the pastoral care of the sick tend to be impoverished by their content. They often focus upon aspects of the illness or "God's will" in such a way as to impose an increase of guilt or lack of responsibility for participating in the illness on the patient. The will of God in these prayers too often appears to be His will for sickness rather than health. Generally, the imagery is somewhat morbid. The real needs of the hospital patient for comfort, presence, peace, and healing are not well defined. For this reason, extemporaneous prayer is most often appropriate to draw together the concerns of the patient and family. Using *their* words from the content of their request further personalizes the prayer. In addition, a corporate prayer draws them further into the relationship of faith and is a reminder of their support and care for one another. These corporate prayers are prayers such as the Lord's Prayer, Hail Mary, or the 23rd Psalm. In this way they gain assurance of their own religious resources.

Healing services, anointing of the sick, laying on of hands have been used since early Christian times in varying forms centered around Holy Communion. The grim aspects of these rites and the impersonal aspects of their prayers have led to their disuse. The Roman Catholic Church has varied them, and uses them now in place of the last rites. The charismatic movement in this country has renewed some aspects of these prayers for healing in their laying on of hands, and this has found ecumenical favor and use. The combination of Holy Communion, Scripture about healings, anointing with oil, and prayer and blessings forms a simple sequence that is appropriate at the bedside. The emphasis is on comfort and healing. However, the patient and the pastor should have a common understanding of what "healing" means in the context of this illness. For some, it would appear, healing is spiritual or even compatible with death. Healing rites should not be allowed to take on aspects of magic or instantaneous gratification with the cancer patient. Although this may occur, it would be most likely after sufficient physical and spiritual medication, the latter based on counseling techniques that encourage a change in the behavior that creates a stressful vulnerability in the patient.

The change in focus of last rites by the Roman Catholic Church is an unfortunate contribution to our cultural denial of death. Both these rites of healing and the dying have a place in pastoral ministry to cancer patients. A prayer that includes a last blessing, a litany for the dying, a form of passage into death and new life is important to many patients and their families, both to personalize and to facilitate their grief process.

A simple outline of prayers for this last blessing might include the Lord's Prayer as an affirmation of corporate worship and individual surrender to God; a prayer that acknowledges the patient as a child of God, member of the covenant, and protected by his might; and a prayer of dismissal. Several Scriptures are suitable for the latter, one of the more appropriate being Luke 2:29-32, the Nunc Dimittis.

The last prayer in the Lucaen passage is particularly effective as a last blessing because it offers to the patient "permission to die." In essence, it is an affirmation by the pastor and the patient that life as they know it is ended. Further, the relationship with God is recalled, and there is assurance that His love will continue even in the confrontation with death. The positive gifts of life are summarized, and the patient's place in the promise of the covenant is affirmed and acknowledged as good. Whatever other prayers are used, they should include these points of reassurance, relationship to God, a summary of life, and an affirmation of God's promises and presence.

MEDITATION

Meditation, in a variety of forms, has become increasingly popular in the last few years. Transcendental meditation and other forms of contemplative prayer are frequently used to relax stress, promote creativity, and improve relationships and self-awareness. Religious meditation has fallen into some disuse. However, the principles are similar and can be helpful to bedridden patients. They have more time to reflect upon the meaning and value of their lives and to discover some different ways of changing them. For the cancer patient whose need is to be in control, the letting go process necessary in meditation often makes him feel too vulnerable. If, however, under pastoral direction, he is able to spend a short period of time in relaxed reflection upon a suitable religious topic, this process can serve as a beginning for more substantial changes later on. Moreover, the short time periods may be lengthened to provide a reduction of stress in the hospital setting. It would seem that appropriate foci for meditation would include positive elements such as healing and the presence of God. Occasional glimpses into the nature and content of the Passion might be suitable, but it would seem that most cancer patients already have a significant and sufficient understanding of what it is to suffer. Short Scripture phrases or even the ejaculatory prayer of Christian mystics, such as "My Lord and My God," are a good beginning. In addition, literature along these lines would be helpful, both as inspiration and as guides.

Reflection and meditation can take many forms. The focus is change and letting go of control. Encouragement to examine one's past life-style, to reflect upon one's gifts without preaching, and to find strength for future change without manipulation requires forbearance on the part of the pastor. Cancer patients who often find change difficult may be reluctant to try new ideas, yet when their old defenses and answers fail to sustain them, the pastor may find opportunity for suggesting some form of meditative prayer.

CHAPTER 5

THE SPIRITUAL JOURNEY

A SPIRITUAL journey is a transcendent process through which we, as human beings, find meaning and value in and for our lives. A spiritual journey takes place concurrently with our physical and emotional maturation, sometimes harmoniously, and sometimes retarded by the adaptations with which we respond to our lives, relationships, and the cultural milieu. The focus for the journey from which all else is circumscribed is our relationship with God. The patient and family's relationship to God, rather than doctrine and dogma, informs the progess of the journey. Different behavior, loving and trusting, is an indicator of forward movement on the journey. The adaptations, cultural, familial, and social, that retard our spiritual growth result in immature religious behavior mistaken for faith, and idolatrous relationships. Spiritual growth may not take place until one is confronted with a crisis, a judgment of one's life and faith. Such a crisis would be the diagnosis of cancer.

The magnitude of the crisis that cancer precipitates in a patient and family unit is inversely proportional to the immaturity of the spiritual progress of these persons. The diagnosis of cancer threatens the patient and family in three ways: first, the prospect of uncontrollable and unpredictable change, including death. The change is ominous, swift, and devastating in its alteration of total life-style, occurring with cancer and its treatment whether or not the disease process ends in death. Second, popular mythology of the cultural milieu believes cancer is synonymous with the biblical leprosy, with painful suffering and/or quick death. Third, the diagnosis itself is received with feelings of judgment. These feelings are often self-inflicted by the patient and family efforts to cope with the reality of the disease process. The patient feels judgment. The underlying problem is the quality of one's life and faith, and the nature of one's relationship to others and to God in the spiritual journey to the present. Generally, the patient's relationship to God is poor, as are interpersonal relationships of the cancer patient.[31] God is seen as detached and punitive in His actions, perhaps a personal projection of the patient or family. Because of this spiritual disorientation and the enormity of personal fears and fantasies about the diagnosis of cancer, the task of coping with the disease and illness seem hopeless. It is this feeling of hopelessness that characterizes the response of many newly diagnosed cancer patients and increases their sense of despair and helplessness.[32]

Movement and growth in an individual's spiritual journey cannot proceed or even begin until the diagnosis of cancer has been accepted openly by both patient and family. Oncologists often will not accept as patients a family unit in which there is secrecy about the diagnosis and treatment. Where there is denial of reality, there is no opportunity for mature spiritual development.

In an effort to maintain control of the situation and to fend off the feelings of helplessness and hopelessness, a patient and family struggle with the reality of the diagnosis. They ask many questions and search for external reasons for their suffering. Generally, this questioning takes place in the past tense, using rational, learned faith answers that seem appropriate to rhetorical questions of suffering and meaning. The medical answers of the treatment process may be used in the same way, and when illness is seen solely as a medical problem with medical answers, the patient and family will search no further for total healing, nor grapple with the spiritual realities.[33]

GOD, WHY ME?

Generally, the discomfort of testing and treatment adds an unavoidable, realistic element to the diagnosis; among the questions the patient and family ask is "Why?," and they almost always include God in this questioning. God still seems remote, but somehow involved in the process of disease, and

---

[31]LeShan, *You Can Fight for Your Life*, p. 65.
[32]LeShan, *You Can Fight for Your Life*, p. 36.
[33]Fairbanks, Rev. Rollin, "Ministry to the Dying," *Journal of Pastoral Care*, 2:9, 1948.

generally perceived as the causitive agent. Blame must be assigned if there is a victim and a rational answer. God is a convenient focus for their anger, guilt, and fear.

The patient and family search their own past, too, for what they have done amiss. Usually they do not have the tools or the insight to discern elements in their life-style that have made them vulnerable participants in the disease process. The idea of their being victimized by cancer and sometimes by God is more acceptable to persons who are all too readily convinced of their worthlessness.[34] The past is sought as a comfort; the patient reminisces about a life that has gone well. This reminiscing differs from the later summing up of life in the preparation for death, although it contains many of the same elements. The difference is mainly in the defensiveness with which the patient justifies his good behavior and desire for health. In the latter period, the patient affirms his goodness (worth) for himself. The affirmation is in the nature of a eulogy, without manipulation, simply a factual, positive summing up of life, the patient's life. Acceptance of the disease and acceptance of the reality of one's finitude and humanity often appear concurrently. God is no longer perceived as remote, uninvolved, or a causative agent of evil. Bargaining with God acknowledges his presence and power, but is still an effort to control the situation. Often, feelings of helplessness and hopelessness that accompany physical illness during treatment are countered by continued efforts to control others, including God, by manipulation, prayers, requests for miracles, and spiritual behavior that depends on the righteousness of others. Failure to accomplish healing by these means may result in a patient's giving up since past religious resources no longer seem effective.

Along with the effort to find a rational answer to the crisis situation, those who are religiously inclined hope for an instant answer — a miracle, a cure. God is perceived as one who can intervene in the natural orders of life to physically heal. Healing is not seen as part of a total life process that the patient shares with God.

Another alternative resulting from an inability to control the present or to resolve conflicts is for patient and families to turn

---

[34]LeShan, *You Can Fight for Your Life*, p. 38.

towards the future in their efforts to avoid coming to grips with suffering in the present.[35] God is recognized as Creator and "willing" this illness; the resultant attitude is resignation: "It's God's Will," or "There must be something God is trying to teach me." Again, the ready answer is an effort to personally redeem the crisis situation. The disease is intellectually accepted; God is tacitly acknowledged, but the emotional levels of the grief process and the faith level of the experience of God must be reached before the spiritual journey can begin, before a decision can be made to "offer up," to surrender the control of one's life to God. The patient and family grasps for the elements of reality that will assist them in their adaptation to their present crisis situation. They may make efforts to assure themselves of their immortality through family, job, or possessions in unique ways. They may explore popular psychological approaches to find an answer. They may continue to look for medical answers. The length of this period in the patient and family's coming to grips with the disease and treatment process (past and future) depends on the severity and treatability of the specific cancer and their resistance to letting go, i.e. giving the control of their situation to God. This last rests upon nature and depth of their trust and faith, their image of and relationship to God. Their search for rational answers leads them to mystery, the power of God, and the answers of faith.

CONVERSION AND ACCEPTANCE

The beginning of the spiritual journey is a surrender, a letting go, which takes place only after acceptance of the disease process; not of life itself, although that may be part of the journey at some point, but of one's fears, preconceptions of the future, and efforts to control one's life, one's family, and one's life-style. There is a sense of omnipotence that evidences itself in cancer patients and family units; a reaction to helplessness that is ultimately counterproductive to both the spiritual journey and the healing process. Willingness to accept the reality of the disease brings with it an openness that may have been

---

[35]Carlozzi, *Death and the Contemporary Man*, p. 35.

hitherto unexperienced by the patient or the family. In their helplessness they need to learn to trust, to change their methods of coping, to find faith that will strengthen them and support them. Rather than being a "victim" of a disease outside themselves, perhaps caused by a God outside their situation, they participate in their healing to the extent that they accept responsibility (not blame) for a life-style that made them vulnerable to disease. They come to recognize God as an agent of healing with them in their situation. Values are reordered, religious resources changed and developed, when possible, and control of one's life focused appropriately with a sense of new meaning.

The process of this change, this conversion, takes place privately, as a rule. After some periods of reflection, patients may share with others the opportunity they have had to take a second look at their lives. There is a summing up, an affirming of all that is good, unlike earlier reminiscing designed to manipulate God into recognition of one's deserved healing.[36]

In the "letting go," which hopefully happens on a spiritual and emotional, and not on a life level, the patient and the family experience new values; different aspects of life are now important to them. They may have desired instant gratification in praying for a miracle, or fantiasized a rapid end to the crisis situation; they may have wished to have things as they were or to hasten the changes that made them so uncomfortable.[37] Having accomplished none of these and finally coping with frustration and helplessness, they settle into the reality of an altered life-style and different feelings about the situation. They experience a renewal of faith in some measure.

MAKE TODAY COUNT

It is often difficult to see this private process taking place. The patients may comment that they live "day by day" and they relate some of whatever has been occupying their thoughts.

Now there is a sense of hope and acceptance, not resignation and despair. The person with cancer is living until he dies, is

---

[36]Carlozzi, *Death and the Contemporary Man*, p. 39.
[37]Carlozzi, *Death and the Contemporary Man*, p. 36.

relatively calm and not depressed about the process, expresses interest in others and their situations appropriately, taking care of his affairs and giving the appearance of having found some new spiritual resources in his life. These resources may include friends and family in whom he can confide, improved relationships with staff, or a renewed look at aspects of religious life that had been neglected. This often takes the form of reading inspirational books, prayer, and attendance at Mass and other worship services. There is no sense in which this behavior is like the religious behavior of those who hope to magically control God. Some conversation about death is often part of facilitating the spiritual journey. Whether the journey will end in death now or later on in life, the encounter and belief about death, as well as experiences of the deaths of others, shape values and personal faith. The ability to trust in God is made more difficult because of the experiences of death. Death is denied to avoid the necessity of reflecting upon or changing personal values.

Most people, when they turn to this contemplation of death and are asked to talk about their ideas, have a profound and straightforward view of what death will be like. A few do not know, others suspect that it will be marred by pain, which it almost never is. Those patients and their families for whom death is familiar do not suffer as much as those for whom the presence of death is dull ache and monumental fear, a secret and a "thief in the night."

The spiritual journey brings about changes in the responses of cancer patients. They are more able to live with the ups and downs of the disease. They have a sense of their common humanity, no longer being victimized. They are more eager to share their lives with others if they can, and they try to establish better relationships than those to which they have been accustomed. The acceptance is mediated in the dialogue with those who share the spiritual journey, affirming them as the worthwhile persons that they are, which is a great need of their personhood.

The guidelines for the spiritual journey are best summarized as follows:

1. A recognition of the cancer crisis as it *is*;

2. An offering to the situation to God, who is recognized as one who can redeeem;
3. A setting to rights one's life, doing that which has been left undone and a renewal of relationships;
4. Continuing to follow these patterns through the ups and downs of the disease;
5. Accepting one's responsibility for participating in the disease process;
6. Continuing (through prayer, meditation and religious resources) to seek a better relationship with God;
7. Sharing one's life (day, week, etc.) with others while caring for one's self;

Cancer patients have the opportunity to participate in living until they die, and with movement on their spiritual journey make that life a fuller, more intense experience than they had in the past.

CHAPTER 6

THE FAMILY OF THE CANCER PATIENT

FAMILY RESPONSE TO THE CRISIS OF CANCER

THE family of a dying or critically ill patient is generally understood to pass through many changes during the process of anticipatory grief. Caring professionals who deal with these families are often puzzled by the variety of responses that they encounter and the difficulties some of these responses can cause. Kubler-Ross notes that: "The families' need will change from the onset of the illness and continue in many forms until long after death has occurred. . . .[The family must] maintain a sound balance between serving the patient and respecting their own needs."[38]

Contemporary family and systems theories describe family interaction in its relationship to the family group and to external circumstances. Most family systems have behavior that guarantees continuity of the system from generation to generation in the interpersonal relationships of its members. It appears to be no accident that cancer strikes more than one member of a family. That member may be systematically predisposed to be emotionally and physically vulnerable to this disease by patterned responses to life, the family and cultural milieu.

Additional insight may be gained through observation of the interaction in the families of cancer patients. Roles and interpersonal patterns indicate that family systems of the cancer patients are, more often than not, closed family systems. This observation may not be taken as a rigid rule, yet further study may well prove it to be the normal description of a cancer patient and family unit. The basic difference between an open and closed family system is the family's response to change; the

---

[38]Kubler-Ross, *On Death and Dying*, p. 141.

other differences are enumerated as follows:

The open family system tends to affirm the self-worth of its members and communicates well among its members. It responds to reality with action, and its members are able to make realistic choices. This family system responds well to change.

A closed family system is based on control in relationships, which is regulated by force; self-worth is secondary to power, and the one with power decides what is right. Change is defended against, and poorly tolerated.[39]

Examination of the personality profiles of cancer patients may indicate, furthermore, that family systems with a tendency to be closed respond in this way to the continual crisis that threaten their balance. One may experience a family system in which there seems to be no space for anyone else; the family is aloof, cold, and preoccupied. This is perhaps the optimun of a closed system. Most families actually interact somewhere in between an open and closed system where a few people are allowed to be a part of, but not to influence, the changes that the crisis creates within the family. Persons with authority, such as the pastor, are likely to function well within this closed system family if the family welcomes him and if the pastor has a good sensitive, relationship with the family.

The family is a unit with an identity of its own. The prospective loss of a member means that the family will never be the same again. The family, as everyone now knows it, is dying too. As the family attempts to cope with the loss not only of a member but also of itself, an important part of its behavior involves the responses it makes to this ultimate change. Among the processes that occur in the family responses in this crisis are (1) an attempt to preserve the continuity of the family interaction; (2) an effort to use its capacity for adaptation in a changing environment, which stands in tension with its need to preserve continuity;[40] (3) realistic approaches to the day-by-day ups and downs of the critically ill.

The synthesis of these processes and the tension involved in

[39]Satir, Virginia, *Peoplemaking* (Palo Alto, California, Science & Behavior Books, Inc., 1972), pp. 113 and ff.

[40]Ackerman, Nathan, *Treating the Troubled Family* (New York, Basic Books, Inc., 1966, pp. 59-60.

maintaining a vital balance are important factors that can affect the outcome of the family's grief process. Its ability to reorganize itself in a healthy way depends upon the extent to which the family disassociates itself from and compensates for the lost member. One author notes that "the intensity of interaction with the deceased before his death seems to be significant . . . in the prediction [and the pastoral assessment] of the type and severity of the grief reaction."[41] The family going through this crisis will evidence visible emotional or physical reactions to the underlying tensions, which may be misunderstood if inappropriately diagnosed. "In the working through of the grief . . . a sense of continity can . . . be restored by disturbing the familiar meanings of life from the relationships in which they are embodied and re-establishing them independent of it."[42] The ways in which the family responds will change as they grieve, but their goals — continuity of interaction and adaptation to change — will not.

The family's responses are those of individuals, which form a cohesive whole. They function as an ego mass (Bowen) using similar defenses, synthesizing and balancing both internal and external stimuli to preserve the family as a unit. The family can, for example, regress to meet a perceived threat and use transference processes to draw in an important surrogate.

Family members have roles that they play in response to the processes that involve them. In acting to preserve continuity, a "historian" recites to the family and resource persons similar incidents of family history and family responses to them. In terms of the family of origin, when encountered in a family regression, the historian cues them to appropriate behavior for the *family*. The historian is the source of the family myths and provides access to the family's past. This person will describe family members who have had cancer or died in other situations, how it happened, and what the family felt or did about this. To do this he must acknowledge some of the reality of the present situation and the seriousness of the event that confronts the family. The historian both preserves continuity and provides evidence of past family ability to cope with and adapt to

---

[41]Marris, *Loss and Change*, p. 42.
[42]Marris, *Loss and Change*, p. 37.

change.

More than one family member may maintain denial for the family unit. This may also be a person who withdraws and/or denies geographically with physical absence or emotionally with drugs and alcohol. The "denier" exerts a certain amount of control over the family response to loss, providing the family with a sense of security, enabling them to function in the present, and focusing at least some of the attention on the problems denial "to get their minds off" the patient. Here is something or someone with which the family has had previous experience; they need not feel so helpless in dealing with this situation.

The "informer," a person whom A. S. Robin Skynner calls the "decider sub-system," serves the welfare of the whole. "These individuals who have ultimate control of the passage of materials and information within the system and across the boundaries with the exterior have control of the system itself."[43] The informer is the family's window to the world; in this situation he may have medical knowledge, and he tells the family what he has learned from resource persons or by observation. The data that the informer presents serve to establish continuity of the family into the present situation and assist them in the beginning to adapt more realistically to change. Both the cancer patient and the family will draw on resource persons in an attempt to preserve family interaction or take surrogate roles that they are not equipped to play. They unconsciously recognize (transference) members of the helping professions and even hospital roommates who will respond to their needs and be drawn into the family dynamic, to be released when the need is changed or fulfilled.

Emotions, too, play a part in the family's efforts to adapt to change and continue its interaction in the present situation. Anger isolates and controls, as does the expression of feelings. Kindness, warmth, and patience draw others into the family life. Mood changes result in a different response from yesterday. Rigidity, a refusal to alter routine, and demands to "do something" are other ways in which the family seeks to defend and

---

[43]Skynner, A. S. Robin, *Systems of Family and Marital Psychotherapy* (New York, Brunner/Mazel, Inc., 1976), p. 20.

control itself, and the situation.

The tension and conflict that the family is experiencing in the working out of these processes are basically healthy. Conflict "is a powerful organizing principle of behavior which simplifies and clarifies immediate purposes."[44] Caught in the multiple demands being made upon it, the family "gets together" to begin to deal with the impending crisis and loss.

The defenses used to preserve continuity may be at variance with those used to assist in adaptation when the family members attempt to predict what will happen. In this they are often encouraged by staff and other concerned persons. They may even create incidents within the institutional milieu to counteract waiting with the unknown and the lack of control that they feel. Sometimes their efforts are oblique, perhaps arising from family myths; often they are obvious efforts, such as room changes or requests for consultations. The family members resort to plans with short-term expectations so that they may have a feeling of accomplishment, a reward for coping with the changes they are undergoing. On the surface much of their behavior may be categorized as denial, yet there seems to be more specific purpose in actions such as prediction, mainly, control of the situation so that the family will not be overwhelmed by the external stimuli as it attempts to cope with the impending loss.

Behind the day-to-day life of the family, we find conflict and tension that emerge ostensibly in a nonspecific manner. Most of what can be seen in the grief process is "dependent upon the family's attitude, awareness, and ability to communicate."[45] As the patient's life draws to a close, these abilities change.

The family members, in an effort to meet the patient's and their own needs, reflect the different elements of the patient's response to the illness as well as their own response to the loss. "The boundaries within the family as a whole mirror that within each individual."[46] This behavior approximates the ego state of narcissistic "mirroring" and is designed as a protection for the family as a whole as well as for the dying member. It

---

[44]Marris, *Loss and Change*, p. 98.
[45]Kubler-Ross, *On Death and Dying*, p. 141.
[46]Skynner, *Systems*, p. 10.

permits the family and its members relief and support from the situation and facilitates them in working through the grief process. If family members wish to deny, they will seek out that member whose role is to deny, and receive affirmation of their view of the present reality. What is perceived to be acceptance of death on the part of the dying family member, and diverse reactions on the part of the family, is actually the family's "mirror" of the dying patient. Ambivalence, often encountered in a family member from day-to-day, is the shifting of the family process of mirroring to meet individual needs within the family. As the family moves through the process, the mirroring effect moves, too. More members will reflect the acceptance with which the family begins to let go of a member, yet there always seems to be just one (the outside hope) who will continue denial to the very end, and perhaps thereafter.

In addition to the mirroring effect, the family uses several other prominent behaviors to facilitate its grieving and defenses. "Role rehearsal," an introjection mechanism, and projection. The patient has one or more "understudies" who will take some place in the family interaction after the loss to maintain the family homeostasis and continuity. They may have already developed some of the behavior characteristics of the dying person, which have been latent and suppressed until now. These become more prominent as they are needed for the reorganization of the family. They may remain only character traits or may result in actual action, such as moving from one place to another, or taking care of a specific family member.

Projection often plays a large part of the family defenses in the beginning and in the end of the illness. From the desire "not to tell" the seriousness of the diagnosis "because *he* is not ready to hear it" to concern for the struggle *"he"* has had, "grief becomes more manageable when it is projected on a social drama to which people can relate their behavior."[47] Family members generally respect projected statements, particularly after the loss, when one member assumes knowledge of the dead person's wishes.

Organization of the family processes, conflicts, and their re-

---

[47]Marris, *Loss and Change*, p. 110.

sponses to impending loss in relation to their reactions to change makes sense of behavior that often seems to have little relevance to the situation of the dying patient. The family purposefully, albeit unconsciously, attempts to survive its loss in ways that will enable it to resurrect, to return to its place in the community again in a new form. It has memories of what it was, and hopes for the future, if it has worked through its grief. It has, perhaps in positive, perhaps in negative ways, recovered its equilibrium from its rending experience with loss and change.

CASE STUDIES OF FAMILY RESPONSES TO CANCER, CHANGE AND CRISIS

As an example of the interaction in a family system that is adjusting to the changes of terminal cancer, the following case study is characteristic of a family's attempts to preserve the continuity of family interaction.

Case Study

The patient is a married, forty-two-year-old woman, an only child, no children, successful newspaper editor, whose cancer of the breast has, in four years, metastasized to her brain. Her family consists of her husband, German born, age forty-three, her mother and father, his mother and sister who came from out of town, and several close friends.

Over the period of three months while the patient was dying, the family interaction caused concern for the pastoral and medical staff. Although the oncology doctor was open and honest about the patient's disease and poor prognosis, when the patient attempted to talk about it with anyone, the husband kissed her, put his hand over her mouth, started talking, or left the room. He (and her parents) were in almost constant attendance in her room. Her mother says that she (the mother) does not express emotion, but the father cries a lot. The husband also does not express emotion, but the patient cries a lot.

The mother-in-law is open and freely expressive of her feelings. The husband's sister and friends are not expressive of their feelings, nor do they allow this in their presence. The entire family, however, despite its behavior, insists on talking openly about the illness. The patient expresses a need to talk to the nurses and/or pastor about her feelings of fear and helplessness at every opportunity. The patient's dependent behavior was very controlling of the family, an interesting contrast to the self-sufficient woman described by her professional colleagues. The family seemed to become more dependent on the staff as the patient deteriorated, but efforts to block communication and maintain a semblance of being in control persisted until she died.

It appears here that the blocking of communication, the tension between expression and suppression of feelings, and the dependent-independent need to maintain control were characteristic of the family as a whole. When one member was open to reality, another evaded it; when the patient died, her husband had gone for a walk and could not be located for two hours.

Efforts to give pastoral care to this family were frustrating, and often frustrated by one or more members. There seemed to be little common ground upon which to relate to them as a whole. They were in the process of disintegration, yet their interaction was an effort to continue their personal relationship patterns as usual and to impede communication of the reality of the patient's impending death.

In this second case study, we see the family members attempting to adapt to the changes that the loss of their mother may bring. They made a good beginning towards grieving. The mother does not die, however, and must be moved to a nursing home, creating a whole new situation for them to cope with: the same family adaptation patterns are also operative.

Case Study

Mrs. H. is a seventy-one-year-old widow whose cancer of the breast has matastasized to the spine. She is hospitalized for a total of ten weeks before she is moved to the nursing home. During this period, she almost dies.

The family consists of one daughter, two sons, all married, one adored grandson, and the adopted children of Mrs. H.'s dead sister, one of whom is a retarded child of age forty with a twin sister who is normal. The patient's continued depression, "wanting to die," has upset the nursing staff and the family. The focal family member appears to be Mrs. H.'s own daughter. Although the sons visit, when they are all together, the daughter steps forward and does most of the talking to the pastor. The family's shocked response to the mother's depressed behavior is evident. The change that causes concern is "she has always taken care of us and now she doesn't seem to care about anything." Dependent upon that care for many reasons, the eldest daughter typifies the family's inability to "let go of her." The "care taking" of the mother, if she goes home, and the retarded adopted daughter have now affected the eldest daughter. She appears to both want and fear this change. "I (the daughter) told her if she came home, she would have to do things my way." The daughter showed good insight into her wishes to have her mother live. In this instance, the mother did recover, due in part to her family's wishes that she live — "little Karl needs her" — and unfinished business in her personal financial planning for the care of her retarded child. She was quite angry because the daughter then put her in a nearby nursing home (perhaps the counterpart of the mother's treatment given to the daughter when she was left as a foster child).

An interesting aspect of both case studies of family interaction and their emphasis on "being in control" is the frequency with which the cancer patient's strength or weakness is described by another family member. Generally, these capacities are determined by the relative lack of dependency and expression of feelings that the cancer patient has. The strong person cares for the rest of the family and "never complains about anything." This person also often protects the family from the facts of the illness, including death. However, patients who are characterized by the family as weak due to their passivity or expression of feelings are often actually very manipulative and controlling.

THOSE LEFT BEHIND

Loss of the strong person, the person upon whom the family has depended for its cohesion, may be somewhat more upsetting than loss of the dependent member. Yet, there is no clearcut pattern to the characterization of the general cancer patient's strength in the family's interaction. Objective observers are most likely to note a shifting and a tension in the dominant member of the family. Perhaps this role and function pattern was characteristic of the family member before the disease crisis. Perhaps it is the result of role changes associated with the progressive disease process. This shifting can make assessment of the family dynamics more difficult for pastoral and, in some instances, medical care. To whose requests does one attend when patient and family are in conflict over sacramental or ethical matters? Rarely do all family members concur on treatment or even timing of sacramental visits such as last rites.

A family that is already in crisis will do what it can to avoid more conflict. Thus, many family responses at this time are defenses designed to avoid rather than work through change. After the death occurs, the family will cling together, as a rule, even though it may have been quite fragmented through the years. Decisions such as postmortem examination, funeral, and burial plans may be delayed until absent members are present.

Although the decision for postmortem examination legally rests on nearest of kin, other family members have positive or negative feelings about this aspect of death, and these feelings are usually expressed. Some guilt often underlies this process, particularly if the decision is to have a postmortem. Usually it is the attending physician's perogative to speak to the family regarding this procedure.

Fantasies, continuing denial, and unconscious wishes, as well as feelings of anger, shape the family response to the request for postmortem examination. The desire to do what is right and in accordance with the deceased's wishes are often reasons given for for having the examination done. Past experiences that center around the deceased "not looking the same" or being "disfigured" generally are reasons given for a negative response. In fact, it would be highly unlikely that most postmortems would cause disfigurement. An answer to "Why did this person die?" sought by both the family and medical staff may be important in relief of guilt over real or fancied neglect of the patient and in preventive medicine for the family history.

Perhaps the most realistic model for family sharing and caring during the days after the death is the orthodox Jewish custom of sitting shiva. The essence of this ritual is the gathering together of family and friends to pray and eat and remember the dead.[48] The comfort of the community in all activities surrounds the bereaved. Much has been written about the American ways of death, yet the common cultural caring present in these traditions allows a much more supportive and realistic coping with bereavement than modern Americans presently experience.

The myriad of decisions that must be made for the funeral are generally accomplished with the help of the pastor, funeral director and, on occasion, supportive family friends. Personalization of the funeral service can be helpful in facilitating grief, and when all is finished, when the extended family may have gone its own way, the pastor needs to keep in touch with the needs of the parish family members to continue in the grief process. How idealistic is it to suggest a pastoral call at three months, six months, and one year to the family? This preventive pastoral care, the opportunity to reminisce and grieve, can relieve so many of the painful left-over feelings that surface at these intervals. Decisions that can be delayed must be looked at objectively with the pastor, and the pastor is better able to assess whether the grief process is "stuck," needing further counseling, or proceeding painfully but normally.

For those who are left behind, feelings of anger, rejection, and guilt often predominate. Expressions such as "I'm happy for him now that he's not suffering" are only partial statements of the family's real feelings. Since death from cancer often, but not always, has been a lingering deterioration, the family has had more opportunity to deal with the impending loss. Never-

---

[48]Gerson, Rabbi Gary S., "The Psychology of Grief and Mourning in Judiasm," *Journal of Religion and Health, 16(4):*260ff, 1977.

theless, there is a difference in dealing with the expected future and the real present. Adjustments that have been begun, changes that were anticipated, are pushed along by the death. The family is restructured in a multitude of ways, and its members often, in a real sense, get to know one another again now that old patterns of interaction are gone.

Lest these patterns be viewed as inconsequential, a family case study may give a clue as to the magnitude and potential of change that occurs due to the loss of the mother.

Case Study

The center of communication for the T. family, a sixty-two-year-old woman, mother of three children, died of cancer of the liver. She relayed details (feelings and facts) about one family member to another. When she died, communication between the father and other family members was minimal. The children felt that they were being left out and ignored by the father, while in fact, communication continued with him as it had for years. It was no longer augmented by the mother, and so it appeared that the communication, and hence the relationship, had decreased. New channels and efforts on the part of all family members was required to re-establish continuity in the family relationships.

Insights into the family process by a pastoral observer may often help the family regain its balance after the loss of one of its members. However, the pastor must take care that his assistance facilitates the family's continuity without his being drawn in to fill the place left by the loss; the pastor remains objective in the bereavement care for the family.

CHAPTER 7

PROBLEM AREAS IN PASTORAL CARE*

DEFENSES AGAINST REALITY

MOST professionals in health care are by now aware of at least one theory of the process of separation, e.g. Kubler-Ross's denial, anger, bargaining, hope, depression, acceptance,[49] that normally accompanies a loss. There are some exceptions to the working through of this process when there has been little attachment to the lost object or when anticipatory grief had been prolonged and involved. At other times, however, a process that in theory is simple and straightforward seems to be blunted and defended against in actuality. Some of these defenses are necessary for a time, even as denial is; others subtly block and impede the process, preventing those who use them from fully experiencing the reality and healthy working through of separation. These defenses seem equally applicable whether they are found in people who have cancer, who are terminally ill, or who have other losses.

WORRY — MORE THAN ANXIETY

The behavior we call "worrying" is an integral part of the defenses that interfere with the working through of the grief process. Worry is a cover and diffusion as well as an outlet for a conglomerate of unacceptable repressed feelings (anger, helplessness, loneliness, despair and pride).[50] A single, nonthreatening aspect of a crisis situation is focused upon, thus permitting repressed feelings about the whole situation to emerge safely as worry. The focus of the "worry" is chosen as

---

*Previously published as "What Will Happen to the Flowers When Winter Comes," *Journal of Religion and Health, 16 (4):, October, 1977. Reprinted by permission of the Journal of Religion and Health.* pp. 326-332.
[49]Kubler-Ross, *On Death and Dying*, p. 235.
[50]Kennedy, Eugene, *On Being a Counselor* (New York, Seabury press, Inc., 1973) pp. 138-139.

the lesser of two evils so that the unacceptable feelings and fears about the situation will not overwhelm the person. Worry serves as a defense against reality and intrapsychic conflict; the latter may include both obsessive and masochistic tendencies. Established interpersonal behavior patterns of self-deprecation and low self-esteem are maintained by worry, while underlying feelings and major concerns such as death are ignored.

Case Study

A seventy-eight-year-old widow, Mrs. M., hospitalized for the repair of a colonic fistula, learned that she would have to have additional surgery the next day. Her distress was shown by her restless hands and tears despite her preoccupation with keeping up a good appearance. Her repeated expressions of worry focused upon having surgery "again at my age." She was unable to clarify what "at my age" meant for her. Her attitudes and behavior were shaped by the opinions of her doctor and a friend, whom she quoted as authorities for her repression of feelings.

Worry is consistent with a need to keep up a good appearance; it is socially acceptable to express worry. The person who worries about any situation has feelings and concerns minimized by standard responses: "Don't worry," "everything will be all right," and other, similar statements. False reassurance makes little of the worrier's view of reality and her place in the situation, reaffirms her sense of helplessness and dependency, and maintains the defenses used by the worrier.[51] Encouragement of independent behavior, real expression of feelings, and clarification of underlying concerns will be difficult, since the worrier uses a response dependent on other authorities that agree with her viewpoint. Worry is a way of appearing to function realistically in a situation while others are encouraged to do something to alleviate the evident distress caused by the worry. Should others attempt and/or succeed in making everything all right, the worrier will simply find a new focus for worry as

---

[51]Kennedy, *On Being A Counselor*, p. 142.

an outlet, however, since the real issues, feelings, and concerns are not dealt with.

REPRESSED ANGER — A DEFENSE
AGAINST LOSS OF CONTROL

The taboo emotion is anger. Although a mature person can distinguish between the wish and the action, in the regressions that accompany illness, *fear* of this overpowering, unacceptable emotion serves to control the expression of angry feelings in ill persons and those who relate to them. The hidden but threatening expression of anger becomes a manipulative method of controlling the patient's environment. The power of this repressed anger lies in fantasy. The anger is tacitly acknowledged, but unexpressed verbally, by the angry patient and those around him.[52] We all shrink from expression that may be self-destructive; it violates our values of life itself. The refusal to express anger at God is equally problematic for pastoral care. Patients fantasize that this expression of anger against God may invite even worse disasters to occur.

Case Study

A sixty-four-year-old service station owner had one eye removed for cancer after consulting with three doctors. He was characterized by the hospital staff as a "good" patient; they noted his cooperative attitude and that he made few demands upon them. Prior to surgery, he had no affect and was euphoric. Afterwards he discussed his situation, saying repeatedly that if he got angry, his "blood pressure would rise" and he "might hemorrhage"; therefore, he would "keep calm and relax, it was a matter of will." He projected all of his feelings, using the word "you." He felt that when he went home, which he wished to delay, things would be "the way they were." He had plans for continuing his activities, which were somewhat realistic, but which changed during the course of the session to ambivalent worries. His inner conflict and fear were revealed by the content of his comments, his restless legs, and rapid-fire

---

[52]Kennedy, *On Being a Counselor*, p. 160.

talking, by which he maintained control of his relationships. Repressed anger limited staff and pastoral relationships with this man. He successfully avoided dealing with his fears and anger about the consequences of his survey, e.g. loss of appearance and limitation of occupational skills, which may have "unmanned" him. Confrontation was made more difficult because the staff was placed in the position of being persons who would not want to harm him by making him angry. He was able to deny all feelings as well as his anger, since he was "not worrying and keeping calm." He described himself as being "resigned," which he would likely remain until he began to express some of his angry feelings in the process of working through his loss.[53] His resignation, in fact, had the quality of depression as he struggled to control his anger post-surgically.

OPTIMISM, HOPE, AND DESPAIR

Since optimism sounds a great deal like hope, we often accept it as such in counseling with the terminally ill. It can be, however, a defense against despair and an alternative to hope, which impedes the working through of the grief process. Optimism expresses the desire "to have things just as they were" without an acknowledgment of the reality of the present illness and life situation. Further, optimism has a single-minded view of what the ill person perceives and wishes as healing — a return to full functioning — getting well is seen as a physical phenomenon only. Hope is most clearly seen in the values it chooses, ultimate values in keeping with the reality of the present situation. "I hope that I won't have to die alone," "I hope that I won't suffer much." It is hope that makes the differences between acceptance and resignation; acceptance includes hope in its accommodation to reality.[54]

Case Study

A sixty-eight-year-old widow with spreading cancer has told

[53]Kennedy, *On Being a Counselor*, p. 168.
[54]Kubler-Ross, *On Death and Dying*, p. 238.

the staff she will be "going home soon." She makes many demands on the staff to "do something." She hates the helplessness she feels "waiting for God to take her." She alternately despairs, does not "want to live like this any longer" and prays optimistically that she will get well and be able to take care of her house and her son once more. She was encouraged to control what of her life she could, such as calling the nurses for herself, talking to visitors and her doctor, and accepting her wish to let go and die.

Optimism seems to compensate for the sense of despair that many persons have when they intuitively realize that the end is near. She had expressed this realization symbolically to the hospital staff when she told them that she would be going home soon. If such direct expressions of feelings were not seen by the staff as negative and evidence of their poor care, optimism would not be needed. There would be no one urging the patient to "cheer up" when the patient does not feel "cheery" if the patient's despair was accepted as normal under the circumstances of impending death.

Hope — real hope — can be a part of the healing process in all illnesses. A cure is a possibility in the future. For the present, not giving in to optimism or despair but living with the illness and seeking new alternatives to the old life-style is possible. Hope can open new doors even as illness has closed old ones. Optimism cannot see new options, but clings to old values and meanings, limiting fulfillment of the ill person who is struggling to adapt to radically changed reality.

GUILT — AMBIVALENCE BETWEEN LOVE AND HATE

The idea that we should not, that we must not, hate is prevalent in our society. Like all negative expressions, hate is an unacceptable emotion. In families undergoing a crisis such as cancer, we often see guilt as the consequence of repressed feelings of hate. The underlying personal dynamics, the infantile belief that wishing a person dead or ill causes death or illness, provides a real but inappropriate source for guilt and is difficult to absolve. Further, we realize intuitively that when a person dies, no further working out of the relationship is possible. Those whom we hate we also love with an equal intensity. The attachment that we lose when a person dies is as great whether or not we had positive or negative feelings towards that person. When the love/hate conflict immobilizes personal functioning, guilt provides an outlet so that these intense feelings can be controlled.[55]

Case Study

A thirty-five-year-old woman came into the office after leaving the bedside of her comatose, terminally ill mother, who had recently taken a turn for the worse. The mother was an alcoholic and the daughter had had a very difficult childhood. She was in conflict about her feelings and her roles as daughter, wife, and mother, and she expressed guilt because she could not do more. Therapy, however, had helped her realize that she was doing her best. She could not acknowledge her feelings of anger and frustration at her mother even when encouraged to do so.

Guilt is often projected onto an honest difficulty, in this instance the inability of the daughter to drive two hours daily to visit her mother. Frequently, members of a family feel guilty when they are not present at the moment of death; they feel that they are missing final words. Often, too, they blame the hospital staff for some incident so that they can manipulate the staff into feeling guilty.

Relationships that spawn hatred and the accompanying guilt are often those of extreme dependency. Real needs, albeit excessive ones, are met in the relationship. When one partner dies, the death can be experienced as a final rejection. This, too, can arouse feelings of guilt that are basically neurotic, i.e. not the result of real and deliberate action. The thought process that is often seen in the ill person as well as the family goes something like this: "I am — or she is — ill. I am being punished. I must have done something awful for this to happen: therefore, I am

---

[55]Kennedy, *On Being a Counselor,* p. 256.

guilty, so I feel that way."

Neurotic guilt used as a defense will not be proportional to the event that occasions it. The person or family who must hide hatred with guilt cannot also express love or be forgiven, since forgiveness includes an element of love. Real healing can occur when the ambivalent feelings, the unacceptable feelings, are allowed to surface and are accepted. Not only does acceptance aid the self-worth and self-esteem of the patient and family, but the grief process is also allowed to continue unimpeded by inappropriate defenses.

THE INFLUENCE OF CONTEMPORARY MEDIA ON PATIENT AND PASTOR

Media, the paperback press and television, have popularized a variety of psychological approaches that are influencing public attitudes towards illness. We will see an increasing number of hospital patients and their families who are learning about wholistic concepts of health as they search for a "cure," quick and sometimes quack methods of easing their burden of illness. Their education about such approaches as the charismatic movement, biofeedback and meditative techniques, Elizabeth Kubler-Ross, and the Twelve Steps of AA provide a challenge to the entire hospital health team, particularly members of the pastoral care disciplines.

In the following four typical patient and family contacts, their immediate needs for help, precipitous self-disclosure, and "different" behavior complicate ministry to them. All of these patient/family units were being treated for cancer. They had been searching for additional resources during the treatment of their disease when they learned about these approaches. In the final case, the patient had already used the program in coping with another physical problem and seemed to adapt more easily to her present illness and hospitalization.

The effective use of any and all of the insights gathered from these approaches hinges upon the patient's acceptance of the reality of his disease. By acceptance is meant that the disease and its treatment are not secrets from the patient or the family, and that their communication is open and honest. The disease is also being treated with appropriate medical management. The family members may or may not have reached the levels of acceptance that the patient must have to use any of these methods, but they should be aware of their use to prevent misunderstandings.

The Charismatic Movement

Religion and spiritual healing are resources often used by those with chronic illness. Patients whose ecumenical religious behavior is oriented towards this fundamentalistic approach may find support and healing resources in the prayers and rituals of their fellowship group.* However, misuse and superstitious belief in the efficacy of prayer and healing rituals can create painful tension and stress in those patients who want so much to be "well."

Case Study

A forty-three-year-old, Roman Catholic housewife with four children has a recurrence of cancer of the breast with metastases to her brain and bone. She wanted "laying on of hands" for healing. Her prayer group indicated that her continued illness was a sign of her lack of faith. She did not accept this, for she felt her children needed her, and she wanted to get well. We discussed various aspects of healing, her feelings about her illness, death, and the charismatic movement, and then she received the "laying on of hands." She returned home with clearer understandings of her relationships, values, and spiritual life.

The dicatomy between the prayer group and the patient and their respective needs ruptured their relationship. The patient felt isolated and guilty because she did not have "enough faith to be healed,"[56] and she was ambivalent about her prayer group's judgmental attitude. These feelings complicated her

---

*See *Healing* by Rev. Francis MacNutt for further discussion.
[56]MacNutt, Rev. Francis, *Healing* (Notre Dame, Indiana, Ave Maria Press, 1974), p. 108.

healing process. Her wish for healing alternated between the hope for a miracle, by which she meant "instant cure," and the expectation of dying soon. She needed active support and affirmation of her emotion and spiritual progress made in dealing with the crisis of her situation. Complying with her request for the laying on of hands was only part of the total counseling process as was helping her find other supportive resources for future use.

Meditation, Biofeedback, and Wholistic Health

These approaches and concepts require the patient's acceptance of his disease and the assistance of helpers trained in the techniques as well as a thorough understanding of the concepts and a belief in their efficacy.

Case Study

An attractive, thirty-six-year-old, married woman returned after a two-year remission of leukemia. She learned about the meditative techniques of Carl Simonton during her first illness. She shared his tapes and articles with a supportive group of her family and staff. She did not feel that hers was the "cancer personality" described by Simonton. She knew that she participated in her illness as well as in her healing, and this idea made her feel somewhat guilty. She found Simonton's technique difficult to use in conjunction with proposed chemotherapy because she had difficulty in accepting the return of the leukemia, and she had financial problems arising from continual illness.

The relatively new use of meditation to reduce stress, the need of the patient to actively participate in the healing, and mental fantasies of the healing process are the principles of Simonton's techniques. They require a commitment of the patient to life and health. As with other patients who use similar biofeedback processes, the pastoral problem centers around the patients' guilt feelings when they blame themselves for causing (rather than participating in) the illness.[57] Life-style or personality dynamics may unconsciously make these patients vulnerable to illness, guilt, and self-blame, which are unnecessarily punitive. Acceptance of the illness, new behavior for coping, and an adjustment to a different life-style are realistic goals for counseling these patients.

The Kubler-Ross Family

This book and its discussion of the dying process has become popular not only within the helping professions[58] but also with persons who are seaching for ways to cope with the dying process and control their immediate crisis situation.

Case Study

A fifty-two-year-old man with two children has a recurrence of his cancer of the colon, which now severely effects his kidneys. Before his present palliative surgery for cancer, he told his wife and doctor that if there was "[new] bad news, [he] didn't want to know it." They, therefore, told him nothing of the new, extensive spread of his disease. While talking to the nursing and pastoral staff, his wife says that she has read Kubler-Ross's book. Her husband is "denying," and she wants "to talk to him about dying, and how much time he has left." She remains calmly in control of her feelings and says that she and her children have accepted his death. Her husband rejects efforts by the staff and his pastor, to discuss dying with him, and upon close scrutiny he appears to have at least moderate acceptance of his disease and simply chooses no longer to dwell on it.

The family used the terminology of the dying process both to maintain their own defenses and to provide a rationale for wishing to communicate more openly with the patient against his expressed wishes. His wife wanted him to have time to "get right with the Lord." Perhaps this was part of her own bar-

---

[57]LeShan, *You Can Fight for Your Life*, p. 57.
[58]Kubler-Ross, *On Death and Dying*, p. 2.

gaining; it did not seem to be a concern to her husband. She intellectualized her part in the process and maintained control and peership with the staff. She could describe her husband's part in the dying process, but she herself was not coping with her own anticipatory grief. The result was staff confusion over her perceptions of her husband's feelings, an overlapping of several counselors' interactions with the family, and a need for the staff to be objective about the various needs of the family members to rely on their own perceptions.

The Twelve Steps of Alcoholic's Anonymous

Living "one day at a time" and "making today count" and life-styles that many cancer patients find to be helpful throughout their diagnosis and treatment. They often arrive at this basis of the AA program by themselves. When they do, their life-styles and comments also have other similarities to the tenets of the AA Twelve Steps, which are of assistance in helping them cope with their disease.[59]

Case Study

An obese, forty-three-year-old housewife has early cancer of the lymph nodes, and finally has a mastectomy. She is a member of Overeaters Anonymous and has been using this program for six months to lose weight. She talks freely about the OA program and easily sees how it can be adapted to help her cope with her present situation. However, while working her program, she frightens her husband by making amends to him (the 6th step). He thinks that she is preparing to die from cancer or surgery, and an explanation of what she is doing becomes necessary. She continued to cope well with her mastectomy and chemotherapy use this program.

This patient already had the tools to assist her in coping with this stressful situation of testing, diagnosis, and surgery. She needed support and reassurance that her assessment of the

---

[59]Alcoholics Anonymous, *The Twelve Stops and the Twelve Traditions* (New York, AA World Services, Inc., 1953), pp. 5-8.

situation and her willingness to take a responsible part in her healing would enable her to live with her disease, "one day at a time." She seemed to feel little guilt, possibly because the program has built-in steps for relief of these feelings as well as the improvement of relationships to provide additional resources for coping.

These encounters present a challenge to pastoral care when families and patients are often more up to date on contemporary developments in professional circles than is the pastor. Underneath, however, they are searching for healing and help in the same way that other families might go from clinic to clinic or try new drugs and therapies. They try in these ways to remain in control of their lives, to find hope and help against the disease process.

An understanding of the common dynamics of these contemporary psychological approaches enables a pastor to assist the patient and the family with the tools they have selected to use. Recognition of the underlying issues also enables the patient and the family to abandon these methods in favor of more traditional supportive counseling if this becomes their need. These common dynamics include the necessity of working through the process of accepting the disease and individual responsibility for taking part in the healing process. The return to health (physical and/or spiritual and emotional) may mean adjustment to a new life-style upon leaving the hospital, acceptance and serenity in spite of considerable pain and suffering, or "living until death." Pastoral care of these challenging family units who have "discovered" these psychological approaches in the cultural milieu depends mostly upon the basics of caring for the very "human" persons confronted with the crisis of illness.

CHAPTER 8

EMOTIONAL PROFILES OF
CANCER PATIENTS

IN the period of the last fifteen years or so there has been an interest in evaluating the psychological processes of the cancer patient. Not only have there been reviews of psychological research dating back to 100 years ago, but there have been numerous personality profiles conducted on cancer patients and their families. In addition, these profiles have been separated into categories for the various kinds of cancer, such as leukemia, breast cancer, etc. These studies provide the pastor with considerable data around which to assess the patient and family who are involved in the cancer crisis and to objectively plan pastoral goals that are appropriate for their psychological and spiritual needs.

Doctors, research teams, and others come to similar conclusions such as those expressed by Carl Simonton.

> We mentally participate in creating our own illnesses, including cancer. It is also my opinion and very well documented that we mentally participate in any form of treatment that we receive and that our mental participation influences the response to that treatment. There is much confusion over the mind-body-spirit inter-relationship, but there is a wealth of information about these relationships and this wholistic approach is the basis of my theories for rehabilitation.[60]

Cancer patients appear to lose their personal integrity and may suffer other losses of vital importance to them as well.

Several authors, most notably LeShan, have observed that individuals who develop cancer, both prior to the development of the disease and after the development of cancer, state that they perceive less closeness to the parents than other disease groups studied, that parent-child relationships were difficult,

---

[60]Simonton, Carl and Simonton, Stephanie, "The Cancer Personality and How to Modify it," Lecture delivered to the annual meeting of the Episcopal Hospitals and Chaplains, March 10, 1975. Published by the Institute of Religion and Health, Chicago, Illinois, 1975, p. 1.

and that loss of an important love object occurred shortly before the development of cancer. This object appears to be of
importance to the patient and one in which the individual is
overly invested to the detriment of his own life and development. When this object is lost, for whatever reason, the individual's feeling response becomes of utmost importance.
Generally, it is a sense of helplessness, hopelessness, and rejection, an experience of being out of control. Depression often
accompanies this helpless feeling. These feelings of hopelessness are carried into the diagnosis and treatment process and
are attitudes that make effective treatment difficult.[61]

In addition, behavior that also causes difficulty for medical
and emotional management is the patient's desire to keep up a
good appearance to be motivated to appear good and less dis-
turbed than he or she really is.[62] Other authors add to this
perception of cancer patients when they note that "cancer patients indeed do repress and deny unpleasant effects, such as
depression, anxiety, hostility or guilt," and that some patients,
such as those with lung cancer, show significantly impaired
emotional outlets.[63]

The inability to express one's emotions as well as the feelings
of rejection caused by loss contribute to a loss of self-esteem in
the cancer patient. These feelings are furthered by psychological or physical losses incurred in treatment, by surgery, or
during chemotherapy.

All of these factors contribute to emotional stress, which
appears to make the patient vulnerable to malignancy. Carl
Simonton defines these characteristics as (1) a great tendency to
hold resentment and a marked inability to forgive; (2) a tendency towards self-pity; (3) a poor ability to develop and maintain meaningful long-term relationships; and (3) a poor ability
to develop and maintain meaningful, long-term relationships;
and (4) a very poor self-image. Coping with life under these
circumstances and with the addition of any crisis apart from

---

[61]Le Shan, Lawrence, "An Emotional Life History Pattern Associated with Neoplastic
Disease," *Annals of the New York Academy of Science*, 1966, pp. 780-793.
[62]Blumberg, E. M., Lung Cancer, Inhalation, and Personality. Abstract, *Psychological
Variables in Human Cancer* (Los Angelos, 1954), p. 30.
[63]Kissen, D. M., Lung Cancer, Inhalation, and Personality, abstract, *Psychosomatic
Aspects of Neoplastic Disease* (Philadelphia, 1964), pp. 3-11.

circumstances and with the addition of any crisis apart from the loss is indeed more than most people can adequately cope with.[64]

Simonton also notes ways of altering these attitudes, which have the potential of helping heal the cancer patient with proper medical management. Some of these factors are built into the discussion of the "Spiritual Journey of the Cancer Patient," chapter 3. A positive attitude, rooted in trust and hope, is perhaps the most important resource a patient, family, and medical staff can have. Hope, however, must be evaluated against the reality that it transcends. It cannot be optimism or it will give way to despair.[65]

A study of patients who have lived longer than the expected norm with their disease describes the psychological differences between this group and others who have died of their disease. On the whole, these patients were revealed from psychological tests to be "scrappy," they refused to give up, and insisted on maintaining normal activities. They had more insight, were more flexible, and were free from overconventionality of behavior. They have a rebellious element that allows them to fight rather than acquiesce when confronted with diagnosis of cancer. Additional qualities discussed by this study include a belief in one's self as having the ability to be successful in coping with and improving upon life, while "living with cancer." Cancer patients also indicate that in the area of psychological control, the more they feel controlled by outside events and people, such as cancer, and medical staff or family, the less they see others as trusting and giving.[66]

These studies provide us with the profile of a person who may be grieving, spiritually impoverished, without hope, and who may not be able to use religious resources on any but the most primitive levels. Pastoral experience with the religious counseling of cancer patients agrees with these facts. A ministry

[64]Simonton, Carl and Simonton, Stephanie, "Belief Systems and Management of the Emotional Aspects of Malignancy," lecture, University of Florida Press, June 14 & 15, 1974, pp. 3-8.
[65]Richardson, Alan (Ed.), *A Theological Word Book of the Bible* (New York, The Macmillan Company, 1950), p. 109.
[66]Simonton, Carl and Simonton, Stephanie, "Psychology of Cancer Patients Who Outlive their Life Expectancies," (Fort Worth, Texas, 1975), p. 3-8.

to cancer patients begins on the level of establishing a trusting relationship in the midst of crisis. This may or may not be possible or bear fruit for some time. The pastor must have those qualities that enhance his vulnerability, openness, and most of all, must be able to endure the sense of helplessness and loss of control that the patient and family convey, as the pastor is included in relationships with them.

EMOTIONAL DYNAMICS IN A TREATMENT PROCESS

Simonton notes that "it is immensely difficult for them to talk about their problems with people. They have got to have a positive base for [for relationships], it is hard for them to share their inner feelings because of this low level of self-esteem".[67] Pastors who have a parochial association with the cancer patient have the possibility of continuing or changing this relationship. They would use a more open, accepting, supportive kind of counseling.

The basic elements of the counseling process that underly Simonton's technique are "caring and sharing";[68] their importance to the pastoral care of the cancer patient as well as their universality in all pastoral care makes their modification an important addition to ministry. The tool that is used in conjunction with these basic counseling elements (and with chemotherapy and medical supervision is "relaxation and mutual imagery."

> A patient can do much more for himself both physically and emotionally than we can do for the outside. There is inherent in the emotion, the process in the mind and the emotion and the soul [strength] that helps a person cope with stress, that helps a person come out of an extremely difficult emotional situation many times a better person. The patients best know the solution to their emotional problems because they have lived them up until then.[69]

The Simonton technique of meditation and relaxation consists of a recommended three times a day regular time period in

---

[67]Simonton, "Belief Systems," p. 5.
[68]Simonton, "The Cancer Personality," p. 10.
[69]Simonton, "The Cancer Personality," p. 10.

which a patient is trained to use a taped, guided meditation. The tape begins by suggesting a relaxation process for the patient's body and then mental imagery of the chemotherapy slowly removing the cancer.* The importance of the patients' using this technique is twofold. First, they willingly take responsibility to do something to help themselves get well. They begin to face the hopelessness and fear that confront them with the diagnosis of cancer. They also use biofeedback principles to combat their fears of continued or recurring cancer.

> A person constantly flashing pictures of new cancers growing in the areas of their body is mentally picturing the worst thing that could possibly happen and that is what goes on in the mind of the cancer patient [and in those who have reoccurred]. It goes on for years until they trust to the fact that the disease will not return.[70]

However simple the above technique appears, a major problem confronting both counselor and patient is the state of hopelessness that pervades by six to eighteen months after the diagnosis of malignancy in a vast majority of cases. Often, hopelessness and general attitudes of fear and bias concerning cancer prevent the patient from trying different forms of treatment and taking responsibility for their healing. Cancer is *the* disease we can do nothing for, and other disease processes appear separated from cancer. If someone says "my doctor told me I have cancer," the immediate thought is, "he is going to die." The cancer patients, their families, friends, neighbors, and professionals around them *expect* and believe that cancer will kill them.

CHANGING ATTITUDES AND BELIEFS

Both Simonton and LeShan comment on the need to change the patient's beliefs and attitudes toward the terminal nature of the disease. LeShan,

> My approach to the terminally ill is oriented toward life and based on the belief that one can search for the fullest use of

---

*Note: This Process should be used in conjunction with medical management and with the assistance of training and therapy at the Simonton's Institute.
[70]Simonton, "The Cancer Personality," p. 9.

oneself under any conditions. If the therapist has unresolved feelings of futility or hopelessness due to the fact that he is working with a dying patient, these feelings are likely to be communicated to the patient.[71]

Simonton uses similar therapeutic changes in beliefs about life in addition to educating his patients to "change their concept of the disease. . . Cancer is not a big problem and that is not a popular concept to hold."[72]

Simonton goes on to describe how this belief change occurs in the patients who come to their institute and use their techniques.

> We get the patient started positively with today. On the basis of day-to-day living, looking at the disease as if they mentally participate in it is a healthier way of living that day . . . the alternative to the here and now of the patient is hopelessness. They do what they can mentally to participate in getting as well as possible. It is easy to delve into why the disease developed . . . to look at the past and find all the things that have produced that state of helplessness and hopelessness one finds in a cancer patient. It's much harder to make today or tomorrow more meaningful.
>
> In addition to the [the relaxation and meditation] in the way of psychological help, they are exposed in therapy sessions to other patients who venture the process, who are turning around their disease so they can talk about their feelings. They can see people who are having some success, they can share ideas and increase their awareness of how their minds and emotions participate in their disease.
>
> The idea of personal responsibility for disease is an idea that has to be handled tactfully with patients. Eventually it occurs to the patients, if they are talking about their cancer, that most of the manifestations they are suffering from are caused by the physiological disease processes of the body. It dawns on them, "if this doctor really believes I can participate mentally and get well, how did I participate mentally in getting sick?"[73]

This insight is a difficult, but crucial turning point in their treatment. First of all, while they bear responsibility in getting

[71]LeShan, *You Can Fight for Your Life*, p. 98.
[72]Simonton, "The Cancer Personality," p. 5.
[73]Simonton, "The Cancer Personality," p. 11.

sick, as opposed to the current attitudes where they are "victims" of cancer, they cannot take blame and need not feel guilty that they have cancer. Too often it is easier for cancer patients to add that guilt to their already negative attitudes towards themselves. Yet Simonton goes on to say,

> A person never wants to die or have cancer, they may have certain needs, crucial needs that are important in living which are not being met, or they may be in a difficult . . . or hopeless situation . . . [and maybe] their minds says cancer would be a way out. We may never know the truth about how much our mind influences our body.[74]

In this crucial time of insight, patients may or may not make the connection between disease process and unmet needs and participation in illness.To encounter the reality of their illness, the patients may need to bring into the open the reality of their lives and their true selves. This last must be accomplished in terms of what is right and positive with the patient as a person, above and beyond the disease. In this way, the insight of personal responsibility and participation in the disease process becomes bearable.

The results of this multidimensional mode of treatment have far-reaching consequences, according to Simonton:

> After the patient begins to use the relaxation and meditation techniques for two or three weeks, regularly; they get some feeling for the process and of their own ability to influence their body. . . . Relaxation will allow the body to get back to its normal state again and energy seems to increase. [Day by day] they feel they have had an influence, they have less pain, they have more energy, and that begins to give them confidence.[75]

At this point, the cancer patients begin in therapy to take what LeShan calls "the third road,"[76] a life-style that may include, but no longer bogs down in, either illness or previous behaviors by seeking out a new and alternative, integrating lifestyle. This must be accomplished within the environment and milieu, the family, job, and relationships in which they live.

---

[74]Simonton, "The Cancer Personality,,' p. 12.
[75]Simonton, "The Cancer Personality," p. 13.
[76]LeShan, *You Can Fight for Your Life*, p. 132.

Simonton feels that it is vital, therefore, that the family be included in the treatment process for this reason.

> A person [cannot be taken] out of their environment, worked with in therapy, put back into their environment and expected to achieve long lasting results . . . the impact and effect of that environment is far greater on that person than the week or 10 days or month [spent with the treatment program].[77]

For this reason, the taking of the third road is an option that requires radical change in some instances. This kind of change is often difficult for cancer patients to make, yet with the support of the pastor and perhaps other counselors and with the involvement of the patient's family, a new life is possible.

---

[77]Simonton, "The Cancer Personality," p. 14.